Don't Kill My Lyme

Don't Kill My Lyme

Just Get Me Better

WYATT PALUMBO

ISBN-13: 9781537732138
ISBN-10: 1537732137
Library of Congress Control Number: 2016916042
CreateSpace Independent Publishing Platform
North Charleston, South Carolina

Contents

Foreword

BY EDWIN JAMES DEAN, MD

Don't Kill My Lyme is a paradigm shift in the approach to treating Lyme disease and other illnesses. Wyatt Palumbo has written a very important book that will make a major impact on the health of many of us and on the way we think about attacking pathogens.

Initially, I was very skeptical when approached with the healing concepts proposed by Wyatt and his Lifestyle Healing Institute philosophy. In my thirty years of practicing medicine, I've spent much of that time as a traditional allopathic physician, which means I mainly treat illnesses once they've manifested themselves. Trained as an emergency medicine physician, I've always been attracted to methods that work and work quickly. I was less interested in the mechanism as long as it's legal, ethical, and it works - even if it means moving from conventional allopathic Western medicine to alternative medicine. Fortunately, I was open minded enough to listen to Wyatt long enough to spark my interest. I was impressed by his knowledge, level of training as a chemical engineer, and experience working in a clinic specializing in drug detox and eventually Lyme disease. I told him if what he proposed was just fifty percent effective, it would help many people, and I agreed to do a few case studies to verify his claims. Our very first patient was a previously highly functioning individual who became debilitated by severe insomnia, anxiety, and abdominal pain. He had gotten to the point where he felt he couldn't continue living life like that anymore, despite having a loving family and successful career. He had seen multiple physicians, psychiatrists, and psychologists and had extensive testing, including CAT scans, colonoscopy, and upper endoscopy. He'd been prescribed numerous antidepressants, antianxiety and sleeping aids, and GI medications with suboptimal improvement. His color was so sallow that we described him as the "walking dead." In just a few days of Lifestyle Healing treatment, his color and his symptoms started to improve, and after a few weeks, he was back to work as a highly functional individual and father, medication and symptom free. Further case studies confirmed the benefits of this healing strategy. The results have been some of the most profound I've seen in over thirty years of practicing medicine.

Through a series of fortunate and unfortunate events, Wyatt learned first-hand that not all organisms affecting our health need to be "killed." As a chemical engineer, he has an analytic and scientific approach to problems. He's also gifted with a photographic memory and strong drive to understand the world around him. While studying chemical engineering, he became ill due to toxin exposure (presumably mold). Conventional medical doctors treated his symptoms of anxiety, insomnia, and abdominal pain with medications but failed to identify and address the underlying toxin problem. Because his symptoms overlapped those of other chronic diseases, he sought treatment in a wellness clinic. Detoxification and targeted nutraceuticals cured his symptoms. As serendipity would have it, he continued to work at the wellness center in the capacity of a researcher, studying patients debilitated by chronic diseases like Lyme. Even though he recovered from his illness, his curiosity led to a specialized microscopic examination of his own blood, which revealed biofilm, parasites, and Lyme. Though he was feeling completely fine, the common line of thinking was that you must eradicate all pathogens from the body for optimal health. A parasite cleanse resulted in a dramatic reduction in biofilm and organisms verified by repeat microscopic examination; however, the effect on his health was catastrophic, resulting in an emergency visit to a hospital's ER, while throwing him back to previous levels of anxiety, insomnia, and abdominal pain with additional symptoms of heart palpitations and arrhythmia.

Another round of detoxification eventually resolved his symptoms. The story could have ended there; however, the young scientist had an aha moment when he questioned why he felt so good, despite having organisms and biofilm, and why he felt so bad after these organisms were dramatically reduced. The parasite cleanse presumably killed many parasites and reduced biofilm, but the release of toxins in a Jarisch-Herxheimer reaction threw him back into his illness. Could it be that a healthy immune system allows the body to coexist with many less virulent pathogens? Fortunately, he was in a position at the clinic to observe many patients who got better with detoxing and healing protocols only to be thrown into shambles once they started killing organisms and busting up biofilm.

Wyatt introduces the concept that killing Lyme and breaking down biofilm fortresses may not be the healthiest strategy and that a healthy immune system allows us to stay healthy and coexist with Lyme. We can see examples of coexistence across the spectrum of organisms that potentially affect our health: bacteria, viruses, fungi, and parasites. In the past, the paradigm was that bacteria (and other organisms) detected in the body were "bad" or benign. More recent studies show that some bacteria are healthy for our bodies, and optimal health depends on them. Case in point is our gastrointestinal biome, which is the diverse collection of bacteria within our gastrointestinal system that helps with digestion and a healthy immune system. The new paradigm is that there are some beneficial bacteria in our bodies that are necessary for our health, and we've evolved to coexist for the benefit of both them and us.

We see a less symbiotic coexistence when it comes to certain viruses. Similar to bacteria, our bodies have apparently evolved to eradicate certain viruses but to coexist with others. To some viruses we have little or no defense, and if infected, we die; an example of this would be the rabies virus. Other viruses, such as the flu virus, can be effectively destroyed by our bodies. Yet there are some viruses that our body can't get rid of completely, and they stay with us for life - oftentimes without any symptoms - if our immune system keeps them battened down, at bay, and hidden in our cells. The herpes virus family is one such group. It includes not only herpes 1 (typically oral cold sores) and herpes 2 (typically genital lesions) but also chicken pox, Epstein-Barr (EBV, the mono virus), and cytomegalovirus (CMV). These viruses never leave the body once infected. Interestingly, most adults show past infection with EBV and CMV; however, they have no history of having mono - myself included. And prior to routine and early childhood vaccination, the same was true with chicken pox. A healthy immune system treats the initial infection, sometimes with minimal symptoms, and suppresses the virus, which retreats to hide from the immune system hidden in the body's cells. They remain there without causing illness as long as the immune system stays healthy. Interestingly, chicken pox virus can explode into shingles or even disseminated chicken pox if the immune system is compromised. Could it be that Lyme and other parasites have a similar course in the body? Initial infection may or may not cause symptoms, depending on the load of infection and the health of the immune system. A strong immune system may knock them out to a large degree. Some survive by creating a fortress of biofilm, not causing any significant health problems until the immune system is compromised.

Wyatt's Lifestyle Healing Institute's philosophy allows the body to heal itself once given the proper tools to boost the immune system. A healthy immune system is key to our health. I was a medical student in New York City at the beginning of the HIV and AIDS epidemic. I realized that once the immune system deteriorated to a certain level in AIDS patients, opportunistic infections started popping up and eventually would run rampant. It's as if there's a great big bacterial, fungal, parasitic, and viral jungle out there, and our bodies are one big petri dish ready to support the growth of these organisms once the immune system gets compromised. What I realized even more was the idea that all of us are exposed to these organisms yet remain disease free, with our immune systems quietly and effectively knocking out and beating back these potential pathogens.

Working with Wyatt has led me to study and question traditional medical dogma. Partly from skepticism and partly from curiosity, and even though I felt healthy, I decided to have a live blood microscopic. It was fascinating to see live white blood cells move across the screen magnified thirty thousand times! While the examiner gave me an A- with regard to my overall assessment, to my astonishment there was evidence of candida, a few parasites, and possibly

Lyme. Until that point I always believed that blood was a sterile environment without any organisms (unless compromised), yet here was my own blood on the big screen with evidence of parasites despite feeling completely healthy. If seeing is believing, what a wake-up call! What a paradigm shift! Could it be possible that the body with a healthy immune system can coexist with less pathogenic organisms and keep them down to harmless bystanders versus having them multiply into an angry and destructive mob? Perhaps similar to most healthy adults, who show past infection of EBV, chicken pox, and CMV however have never had significant related illnesses, I, too, was coexisting with a few parasites and yeast yet never had significant illness. And what if I was to nuke these bystander organisms with antibiotics or with other destructive methods, in an attempt to rid them from my healthy body? Would a Jarisch-Herxheimer reaction lead to a cascade of toxic events and deterioration to my health and well-being? Or would be a better approach be to keep the brain, gastrointestinal, and immune systems functioning at peak performance and allow them to keep the onslaught of pathogens at bay?

You can decide after reading this book. As for me, please don't kill my Lyme.

Introduction

Is Lyme Really Causing My Symptoms?

How do you end up with a diagnosis of Lyme disease? How do people end up with any chronic disease diagnosis, for that matter?

You seek a diagnosis because you don't feel well. You want an answer for why you feel the way you do. You want an answer because it will finally serve as a basis for treatment, a basis to get you better.

No one can blame you for this. It's understandable.

But if you felt better, you wouldn't be looking, you wouldn't be going to doctors, and you wouldn't be seeking answers because you wouldn't be "sick."

You end up with a diagnosis of Lyme disease only because, despite years of effort, years of failed treatments, years of doctors, and years of suffering, you still don't feel well. Lyme finally feels like an answer that can explain what you've been going through for a long time.

For some, a Lyme diagnosis is relief from a long fought battle against the unknown. For others, it doesn't provide a solution; it merely adds more questions.

At Lifestyle Healing Institute, we are usually the last stop for Lyme individuals. I can't tell you how many people have said, "If you can't help, this will be it for me." When I first speak to these individuals, it's horrible to hear how alone they feel. Many have become hopeless, afraid of the disease, and afraid of the future; they're afraid they're going to feel this way forever.

How does someone get to that point?

Most of your initial health issues leading to the progression of chronic Lyme are due to the very physicians who are treating you. American medicine falls short when it comes to the treatment of chronic disorders. Many of you will present with a relatively minor issue or symptom such as joint pain, fatigue, muscle weakness, concussion/brain injury, irritable bowel (GI issues), mood changes, anxiety, sleep issues, and more.

What happens next? Your physician fails to treat these issues appropriately, and since you don't get better, you seek another physician, another diagnosis. If you're suffering from mental health issues such as depression, anxiety, and insomnia (common symptoms associated with Lyme), now it's time to start antidepressants, benzodiazepines, and sleep aids. The medical field is failing you and far too many other people. I believe there's a time and a place for everything, but many drugs, especially the ones used in Lyme disease treatment, aren't designed for long-term use.

You went to the doctor because you had some sleep issues, you were stressed out, or you had some uneasiness in your stomach; you wanted some help because you just didn't feel right. Your initial doctor visit is largely responsible for your Lyme diagnosis; your initial physician failed you. Now you're moving from physician to physician, hoping to get some answers. Meanwhile, as time passes by, your fatigue becomes chronic fatigue, your muscle/joint pain and weakness become fibromyalgia and/or chronic pain, your sleep issues become insomnia, your depression makes it nearly impossible to get through the day, and your anxiety makes you feel as if your brain were on fire, as if you were plugged into an electrical outlet. Not only are your original symptoms unresolved, but they've worsened, and now you have a laundry list of new symptoms to accompany them. You still don't feel well; you still don't feel like yourself.

It becomes such a struggle; your disease becomes an act of desperation. Every day is a battle; you can no longer exercise, you might be out of work, and you might find it difficult just to get out of bed, to get through the day.

You eat gluten free and even dairy free, yet you still don't feel as if you're making any strides toward getting your life back. You're online, researching all the time - on Lyme blogs, clinic websites, anywhere and everywhere - just to find some answers. Whether it's through your own research or finally through a physician's diagnosis, you end up with the answer: Lyme disease.

After years of battling thirty or more different symptoms, you still don't feel better. You're slipping more and more each day, month, and year until you finally arrive at a diagnosis of Lyme disease.

Lyme is basically an umbrella description. It's easy to hold on to this answer because of its ability to explain so many of your symptoms. Lyme is one of the only diagnoses that spans across all your symptoms; it makes much more sense than other potential causes you've been diagnosed with. Everything is beginning to click in your head. And hey, if you kill it, all those symptoms will go away, right? (I don't think so!)

Well, now it's time to find a Lyme center. You must kill your Lyme, right?

After you kill it, your body will heal, right?

There won't be any residual damage or worsening of symptoms, right?

I'm sorry, but this is just not true in the majority of chronic Lyme individuals. Even so, to undergo any treatment for Lyme, you must protect the brain and body. If you are fortunate enough not to be on drugs yet, you probably will be now. Whether it's megadoses of vitamin C, hydrogen peroxide, ozone therapy, ultraviolet blood irradiation, herbs, essential oils, colloidal silver, oral or intravenous antibiotics for months or even years, or any combination of the above and more, an experienced physician will probably put you on prescription medications throughout the long, drawn-out months or even years of ensuing Lyme treatment.

"Why?" you ask.

Because your physician knows he or she has to protect your brain and body for what's about to come: an onslaught. You must understand that your symptoms will worsen through Lyme treatment because of what many call "die-off" (a Jarisch-Herxheimer reaction [JHRxn] or a "Herx"). If you were fortunate enough to receive a negative Lyme test (which doesn't mean you killed all your Lyme, anyway), you're now left with tremendous worsening of your symptoms. That's OK because now it's time to rest and let your body heal. If your physician doesn't understand that Lyme is a multifaceted, multifactorial disease, a disease that requires multiple tools across multiple brain and bodily systems to truly heal, do you think they will understand how to help you heal after a worsening of symptoms?

And yes, I understand some Lyme individuals do get better by attempting to kill the disease, and that's great because the goal is and always will be to get you better. Some will be angry and disagree with my notions of Lyme disease, and that's OK too. I wrote this book to give people another way to battle this disease, a way that's the exact opposite of every approach you've tried. Other treatments are merely different ways of trying to kill Lyme. Our method is based on the very premise that you don't have to kill Lyme to feel better, and this proves to be true for our individuals time and time again. The reality is that Lyme is rarely the cause of your symptoms. I realize it's difficult for you to come to grips with that conclusion, especially if you're currently suffering from Lyme, but I will spend this entire book outlining the science, the reasoning, and the proof behind my concepts.

What is inarguable is that Lyme crosses into multiple brain and bodily systems; thus, subsequent treatment must reflect that fact. All treatment for chronic disease must be multifaceted to give you the best chance to heal. You must understand beyond what each of these approaches is and how to use each modality; you have to understand how all these modalities are interwoven and how they relate to one another. Today's treatment for chronic Lyme doesn't reflect this notion. I'm writing this book to provide you with a better way; a more efficient way; a more scientific way; and most important, a way that's different, holistic, and integrative; without the use of pharmaceutical drugs: a way that gets you better.

Yes, I'll present a whole lot of science and data from real individuals showing what happens when you attempt to kill Lyme and why your symptoms worsen, and I'll also explain the need for and importance of a multifaceted approach backed by documented research.

But I also know about Lyme and chronic disease because I've lived through it.

The worst question you can ask someone with a chronic disease like Lyme is "How are you doing?"

I used to hate that question so much because the answer was always the same: "I'm doing bad; nothing has changed." When you suffer from a disease like Lyme, it's either bad, less bad, or extremely bad. There are only degrees of bad; there's no good anymore. You've probably forgotten what it's like to feel good, to feel happy. I know what this is like.

I struggled significantly with depression, anxiety, insomnia, and irritable bowel syndrome when I was in my first year of college. I had a colonoscopy one month into my first semester after I lost seventeen pounds in three weeks (and I'm a pretty thin dude). I got sick once a month, like clockwork, taking antibiotics like candy to get rid of my recurring infections. One month, I got the swine flu; then the month after, I got the regular flu. I finally went to my primary care physician, as I felt as if stress was consuming me, and he gave me Lexapro*, an SSRI antidepressant. Three weeks later, I was suicidal and was referred to one of my university's psychiatrists. She switched me to Zoloft*. (Another SSRI antidepressant—brilliant, right?) Nothing changed, so she switched me to Depakote*, which meant I had to get blood tests to ensure that my body was handling the medication, and it was not causing toxicity. That didn't work, either, so I was given Ambien*, then Ativan*, then Klonopin*. No success. Meanwhile, I spent days without sleeping, I was throwing up after every meal, and my anxiety was so bad it was pretty hard to get through the day. I was then told I was bipolar; that makes sense (not really), as if you could catch bipolar like a cold or something. The bipolar medications didn't work either, so I had a meeting with all four psychiatrists the school had on staff, at which they asked me many questions, trying to determine what was happening. I was even told by one of the psychiatrists that I was a drug addict, and that was the source of all my problems. (She later couldn't face me when I went back to tell them how I actually did get better.) I then switched care to a nurse practitioner, who put me on Cymbalta* and Trazodone*. She was convinced that would do it. Nope.

Months had passed, and I was much worse than when I originally went in for help. Long story short, I ended up seeing seven doctors, with a trial of thirteen prescription medications.

Finally, my dad found a place for me to go that seemed to make sense. The doctor there used a scientific approach, which resonated with me. He prescribed me two more medications to help with my depression and insomnia and numerous supplements to help me with my gut. I can tell you that those medications pulled me out of my hole - my six-foot hole - but when I was done with the treatment, I was left addicted to the medications. I never blamed any of those physicians for what happened to me, because they truly thought they knew what they were doing, though their approaches lacked any sound scientific basis and many were just outright shortsighted.

Anyway, two years later, I researched toxicity and potential infections. I had my biofilm examined and saw massive creatures roaming around in my blood. I had to kill them, right? I went after them hard and ended up in the hospital with a heart arrhythmia. I was then prescribed two more medications to help with my heart and to combat my new symptoms, because I thought I had to kill the infections to kill Lyme. Now I was taking four medications, which helped resolve my short-term issues, but I knew I'd never get to where I wanted to be without getting off those drugs.

I would never tell you I know exactly how you feel, but I can say I've been there; I understand the process you must deal with. I know what it feels like to want to give up, to realize your physicians are grasping at straws, and to know you've got no other choice but to do what they say. Most importantly, I made it through that ordeal, and I'm healthier than I've ever been. I've been prescribed multiple medications, and I have figured out a safe process by which to stop taking them. We can get you better, together. I've used my own struggles to help others and to help you. I've set up our clinic with you in mind. I try to limit my use of the word "patient" because you're a person, an individual; you're struggling, and you need help. I've never understood the saying "If I've helped one individual, changed one life, then I've done my part." That's great and all, but I got into this to help as many people as possible, one at a time, and I won't stop until I reach you. I didn't get into this for just someone; I got into this for everyone. My method and system didn't work just for me; they've worked for numerous individuals, some of whom had nasty cases of Lyme.

This book will show you science, sound reasoning, and real data from people who suffered from Lyme. I'll show you a better way - a way without drugs, a way without painful symptoms, and a way that gets you better without ever treating your Lyme.

At Lifestyle Healing Institute, we help explain the myriad of symptoms you may have, but there's no denying that not one Lyme individual presents with just Lyme. Lyme is merely the catchall diagnosis that helps explain why you're feeling terrible. Nowadays, many people go to the doctor looking for one answer to explain numerous symptoms; they want one thing to "fix" those numerous symptoms; and oh, they wanted it to work yesterday. This is, in part, the American mind-set, so you can't go blaming the pharmaceutical companies (for everything) for meeting this need. Today's traditional allopathic medical practice fails to employ the concepts, science, and fundamental aspects that truly get people better.

I want you to know that there is another way, but I also want you to understand Lyme through and through. The fear of Lyme comes from the fear of the unknown, the fear of not understanding this disease. This book gives you an abundant amount of knowledge about Lyme disease, so even if you choose a different method or clinic, you will feel confident with your new understanding when talking with other physicians. They will not be able to dictate your treatment without scientific and sound reasoning.

The frustration I've portrayed throughout this book, is directed toward the Lyme physicians who don't know how to treat Lyme effectively. This book is written for you, and any sarcasm or frustration isn't directed toward you. I never mean to come across as talking down to you, and I want you to realize my intensions as you continue reading this book. My dissatisfaction stems from my annoyance with the very physicians that messed up the outlook of treating Lyme. Physicians are failing you, hurting you, and I won't watch this happen anymore. When I say you "need" to understand something, I believe it to be an important concept which will help your healing process. That's what I care about – I care about you.

It's important to understand these new concepts and my documented rationale behind the treatment protocols. A needed change in approaching Lyme is now possible because you will be empowered with a vast amount of knowledge concerning Lyme. You will be able to help yourself or seek the correct care that will enable you to heal. I hope that you will share in my passion, and together we will provoke change. It's my passion to help you, to give you as much information and knowledge about this disease. It's important that you know this as you move forward reading this book. With knowledge comes understanding. I want you to understand Lyme.

No disease is just one thing, one answer, and Lyme is no different.

Lyme requires an extensive understanding of the brain, the immune system, toxicity, the food we eat, circulation, the gut, and every other bodily function. Lyme must be treated from top to bottom and from every angle possible, and you must understand how these angles interact with one another. With Lyme, if you treat symptoms or bodily systems individually, one at a time, you are highly unlikely to see any results. You're just not going to gain enough ground to alleviate symptoms, to feel better. The body doesn't function as a collection of separate systems; it functions as one unit. Through this approach, we've gotten numerous individuals better without ever killing Lyme disease. More importantly, Lyme disease is better explained by imbalances, deficiencies, and abnormalities in the brain and bodily systems associated with it. This is crucial in understanding how to successfully treat Lyme. I'm not a fan of using the word *cure*, but if you truly want to heal from Lyme, if you truly want to get better, you must understand that Lyme is rarely the cause of your symptoms.

Simply said, the cure for Lyme disease is understanding that it's not Lyme disease.

When it comes to Lyme, your physician should understand your numerous symptoms and, more importantly, which symptoms point to which causes. Most of you are currently undergoing treatment, and I want you to ask yourself these questions. (For your previous treatments, replace the word *does* with *did*.)

Does your physician understand the brain?

Does your physician understand the mind-body, mental-emotional connection?

Does your physician understand blood flow?

Does your physician understand biofilms?

Does your physician understand the hormonal system?

Does your physician understand immunity and autoimmunity?

Does your physician understand the gut?

Does your physician understand environmental toxicity?

Does your physician understand genetics?

Does your physician understand medications and pharmaceutical detoxification?

I could go on, but I'm sure you get the point.

It's one thing for me to say, "Don't treat Lyme by trying to kill it"; it's another thing for you to understand the basic concepts in treating Lyme and whether your physician is even capable of treating the disease. Let me be clear: Lyme- and all chronic diseases, for that matter - **requires an understanding of and expertise in all bodily systems and more**. Don't let any specialist tell you otherwise. Don't let some specialist put you on antibiotics and tell you that once you've finished the antibiotic cocktail, your Lyme will be gone and everything will be fine.

If you heal the brain, gut, and immune system successfully, you don't have to kill Lyme.

You don't have to kill Lyme to get your life back.

You don't have to kill Lyme to feel better.

You get better by healing the multiple brain and bodily systems exhibiting symptoms associated with Lyme without having to undergo treatment for the disease itself.

It's OK if you don't believe me (at least not yet), because this entire book will explain why it's true.

I just want you to know there's another way, a completely different approach to battling this debilitating disease.

I provide you with scientific research, sound reasoning, and quantitative data from real individuals showing why you shouldn't kill Lyme and, more importantly, how we can get you better without ever killing your Lyme.

Throughout this book, I'll show you how Lyme - and any disease, for that matter - is complex and thus requires a complex system consisting of multiple tools to truly get you better. As I've stated, it requires an understanding of not only how each system works but also how each system is related to the others. You can't have a change in one system and not expect it to affect the whole body; everything is interconnected. It doesn't make sense to expect to kill your Lyme and suddenly have all your symptoms go away, yet this is what many believe and pursue. This results in long, drawn-out, debilitating Lyme treatments, yet Lyme by itself is only the spark that started the fire of body dysfunction. To squelch that spark and not address the ensuing and ongoing fire misses the mark.

Don't your brain and brain-chemistry imbalances play a role?

What about your hormones? Don't they contribute to your symptoms?

What about immune dysfunction?

How about circulation and blood-flow abnormalities?

What about the gut and malabsorption?

Don't your mind and mental-emotional disturbances play a significant role?

Everyone who has Lyme has excess inflammation and environmental/industrial toxicity, so what about those?

The bottom line is that each of these systems and conditions play a role in causing your symptoms. More importantly, you'll find that disruptions in these systems explain your symptoms much more accurately than Lyme itself. You'll realize they're the true causes of your symptoms and not Lyme disease, the spark that started the fire of dysfunction and, subsequently, your symptoms.

Our bodies are extremely sophisticated and are undoubtedly our most efficient healing tools. We'll provide your body with what's needed to achieve both short-term and long-term healing. You can't successfully treat Lyme and get people better without addressing the subsequent dysfunction in multiple body systems. Although many disagree, it's an absolute impossibility to tie all your symptoms back to Lyme. You'll find your Lyme alone is rarely the cause of any of your symptoms.

When there are various disturbances in our bodies - whether toxins, pathogens, emotional disturbances, or something else - our bodies compensate. However, when these disturbances aren't resolved, the compensation mechanisms become exhausted, and the brain and body begin to break down. As our bodies begin to break down and become depleted, we become vulnerable to more disturbances, to more disorder, and to more damage. As our bodies become more and more depleted, the damage, which includes brain imbalances, immune dysfunction, hormonal suppression, blood-flow/circulation abnormalities, GI issues, and more, begins to take a major toll on the brain and body.

Most, if not all, of these conditions must exist to provide a platform, an environment, for your Lyme to even cause symptoms at all. To get you to understand my point of view, I'll go into detail about the overwhelming damage to the brain and body when individuals undergo Lyme treatment. I'll then show you how we heal your body without your ever having to endure the draining process of treating Lyme disease. More importantly, your symptoms are a result of these interacting disturbances, not Lyme itself. Treating these disturbances and understanding the complexity of each of their roles are the keys to getting you better safely and in far less time.

One

A Brief Understanding

As a society, we've been fighting for virtually all our human existence. This fight has carried over to medicine because we want to kill any foreign invading pathogen, without much concern for all the collateral damage. This collateral damage causes more issues than the Lyme itself. The only difference among various Lyme treatments is how to kill the disease; in the end, these approaches aren't really that different from one another. It's not uncommon for individuals receiving treatment for Lyme to end up on multiple prescription medications to resolve misinterpreted symptoms. Your physicians don't know how to manage your symptoms or how to treat your Lyme; they may have your best interest at heart, but many only make you feel worse.

I'll show you another way, a much better way. We replenish, restore, revitalize, and reinvigorate your body, allowing it to do what it was designed to do. The mentality of supporting all that's good in the body and stopping our conditioned war-and-destroy mentality has been gaining speed in recent years. For example, this philosophy is seen in gut health in the use of probiotics, which use beneficial bacteria to restore gut integrity and reduce harmful bacteria - hence, supporting the good to overcome the bad. But this approach hasn't carried over to other conditions, especially when it comes to common infectious diseases like Lyme. This philosophy is what's needed to appropriately treat Lyme, and when treatment is done properly, it results in far less treatment time without the use of pharmaceutical medications.

As you may already know (but in case you don't, I'll explain it later), Lyme builds a biofilm: a protective fort that shields the disease from most of your own defense system, your immune system. A biofilm is impervious to many common killing tools, especially antibiotics. You'll see how ineffective and outright dangerous the use of antibiotics is in treating Lyme and any other disease that builds a biofilm (which accounts for 80 percent of infectious diseases).

Biofilms' ability to adapt and survive far supersedes ours. They've been around for 4.5 billion years. The same biofilms that house Lyme also contain toxins, fungi, candida, coinfections, and more. To kill Lyme, you must breach the biofilm. As you've probably experienced, when you do this, your symptoms worsen, new symptoms develop, and you're no closer to eradicating Lyme. The terrible symptoms associated with killing pathogens like Lyme (commonly known as a Jarisch-Herxheimer reaction) stem from everything that's hiding within the biofilm. In terms of any biofilm-based disease, a treatment that results in breaching the biofilm causes a Jarisch-Herxheimer reaction far different and far worse than originally proposed by Adolf Jarisch and Karl Herxheimer themselves. Lyme proves to be insignificant in comparison to the debilitating results after the biofilm floodgates open upon breaching.

Is all this really necessary?

Is killing Lyme necessary to feel better?

Throughout this book, you'll see why it's not necessary. You'll see how and why a multitool approach to healing is the best way to heal Lyme or any chronic disease, for that matter. You'll see our healing program is done without the use of pharmaceutical medications. You'll realize there's another way. You'll realize you'll get better without ever killing your Lyme.

What Is Lyme, Anyway?

One of the most common questions Lyme individuals have after their initial diagnosis is "What do I do now?" To answer that question, I should delve into everything that relates to Lyme: your symptoms; other related diseases; how a diagnosis is reached; and most importantly, how we get you better. But first, I want to explain how we got to this position and provide some clarity on common misconceptions regarding Lyme.

Let me start by explaining a few basic concepts regarding any pathogen. Pathogens, which I'll be talking about frequently, are entities that cause infection in humans, such as bacteria, parasites, and viruses. Lyme is a type of pathogen, as are many coinfections associated with Lyme, such as bartonella, babesia, and mycoplasma. Viruses, such as HIV, herpes, and hepatitis, are also pathogens. They are all entities that frequently cause infections in humans.

There are two kinds of invasive pathogens that disrupt the human brain and body. One type we are much more familiar with. These are pathogens that attempt to enter our bodies and cause havoc by releasing signals and toxins to disturb the innate balance in our bodies. Many disrupt and even inactivate our immune systems (our defense systems), like many common bacterial infections, some viruses, and cancer. The second type is a much different breed, a sort of stealth invader that hides from your immune system in an extremely systematic and sophisticated way. Lyme is of this different breed of pathogen, which our world is just beginning to understand.

I know you're interested in how to heal from Lyme disease, and I'll explain my process, but first I want to show you how we got in the predicament of this pesky stealth-infection era. If you can't wait, go to the table of contents and flip to whatever page you'd like, but be sure to come back and read this later. First off, here are a couple of paragraphs on the history of the discovery of Lyme, and yes, there is a point to them, so you should read them.

In 1981, a scientist named Willy Burgdorfer found that the connection between Rocky Mountain spotted fever (caused by a tick bite) and Lyme disease was a bacterium called a spirochete that was causing Lyme: thus, the name *Borrelia burgdorferi* (the fancy scientific term for Lyme). Willy

Burgdorfer credits Dr. Sven Hellerstrom with the initial discovery of Lyme in 1949 when he discussed a paper presented at the forty-third annual meeting of the Southern Medical Association. This is where Hellerstrom discussed the discovery of erythema chronicum migrans (ECM, a type of skin lesion) and Lyme disease. Documented history of erythema migrans dates back many years, but in 1909 Arvid Afzelius described a case of a skin lesion at a dermatologic meeting in Sweden and thought the eruption was likely produced by the bite of a tick. The initial description of Lyme arthritis appeared in 1977, with patients describing a rash thought to be erythema migrans (1, 2).

In the late 1960s, Dr. Rudolph J. Scrimenti treated an ECM patient based on the detailed description of the patient's tick bite preceding the illness. Remembering the success that the Swedes had had with penicillin treatment, he treated the fifty-seven-year-old patient with penicillin; he was symptom free in a short time and remained that way until his death twenty years later. ECM was called "Lyme arthritis" in Europe and was often curable if treated immediately with penicillin (2).

In the 1970s, in Lyme, Connecticut, children and adults suffering from symptoms that included swollen knees, paralysis, skin rashes, headaches, and chronic fatigue were left undiagnosed until the medical establishment studied their symptoms and finally surmised that they all had been bitten by a tick in the same region. Researchers named the syndrome - you guessed it - Lyme (2). The first case of Lyme was found in a five-thousand-year-old mummified individual. No surprise there, as biofilm-producing species, like Lyme, have been around for 4.5 billion years.

Fast-forward to today, and forty years after Willy Burgdorfer was credited with its initial discovery, research into the causes of posttreatment Lyme disease syndrome (also known as chronic Lyme disease, which is what I call it throughout this book) has a home at the Johns Hopkins Lyme Disease Clinical Research Center, which opened in 2015, supported by a gift from the Lyme Disease Research Foundation. **Lyme is now the sixth most common reportable infectious disease in the United States**, costing the economy $1.3 billion per year (3). Many feel it's becoming an epidemic and one of the most debilitating diseases of the Western world.

In 2012, Lyme disease was included in the top ten notifiable diseases by the Centers for Disease Control and Prevention (CDC) (4).

In 2013, the CDC reported more than three hundred thousand new cases of Lyme disease each year in all states except Hawaii (5).

Now to my point: the underlying theme of medicine in the mid-1900s was the discovery and use of antibiotics. When Lyme was initially found, it was treated with antibiotics. In modern medical society, bacterial infections are treated with antibiotics, and Lyme is still no exception. Therefore, it makes sense that even today, Lyme is still treated with antibiotics.

However, over the past sixty to seventy years, in response to our use of antibiotics, invasive pathogens have developed new maneuvers; they've become smarter because of our everlasting pursuit of eradicating them. Infections that are not easily eradicated using antibiotics are now posing a much larger threat than ever before. These infections are usually biofilm-producing infections, and instead of going after our immune systems directly, they just hide from us in a nice, cozy fort with their friends, safe from the onslaught of our immune systems. If you attack them with antibiotics, they become even more resistant to any subsequent therapy. (Biofilms are discussed in much more detail in Section 2.) The National Institutes of Health (NHI) estimates that 80 percent of all infections build biofilms (6). This means that our approach to infections for 80 percent of infectious diseases must use a different approach that doesn't involve antibiotics. It's becoming impossible to ignore the role biofilms play in current medicine. Lyme falls into the 80 percent of infectious diseases that build a biofilm (7).

It's estimated that only about 10 percent of individuals see the infamous "bull's-eye" rash; thus, only 10 percent of people know they have Lyme at the time of infection (10). These 10 percent, if treated within the first two weeks, can sometimes successfully eradicate Lyme using antibiotics.

Why is Lyme easier to handle in those 10 percent?

Because Lyme hasn't built its fort yet. It hasn't built its biofilm fortress.

What's so special about biofilms?

Biofilms are unaffected from using antibiotics. They render antibiotics completely ineffective, which is quite dangerous. Many may disagree, but these are the facts: "To date no antibiotic treatment exists for biofilm formation" (8). I'll explain why and how and provide significantly more research in Section 2, "Biofilms."

So, if you've been keeping track of the math, that leaves 90 percent of Lyme-affected individuals not knowing they have Lyme, which means they've got a fortress on their hands—more importantly, a fortress highly impenetrable by antibiotics.

It's interesting because there is a term for that 90 percent: it's called chronic Lyme disease or posttreatment Lyme disease syndrome. I don't understand why the minority (the bull's-eye 10 percent) gets the clean title of Lyme disease, and the majority (the other 90 percent) gets the more complicated title. But getting into the realm of how certain syndromes and disorders obtain such interesting names is a discussion for another day. Just ask the innovators of the ICD-10; I'm sure they'll be able to help you out with that one. (The ICD-10 is the tenth revision of the International Statistical Classification of Diseases.)

Throughout this book, I will be using the term *chronic Lyme* often. When I say *chronic Lyme*, I am referring to the 90 percent of Lyme individuals who do not get the bull's-eye rash and are unaware they have the disease for weeks, months, or even years after the initial infection.

Simply said, this book is about the 90 percent of Lyme individuals for whom traditional treatment has failed, those who are looking for a better, scientifically researched, more all-natural and integrative approach to healing (chronic) Lyme disease and everything that comes with it.

Chronic Lyme Disease According to the CDC

I have my own opinions on Lyme and various other chronic diseases, but if I can't back them with sound reasoning and science, I tend not to share them. I've read numerous opinions, some of which I agree with, some of which I do not. In the end, I don't want to give you a blanket statement without facts and sound reasoning, even if I'm convinced of its validity. With that said, I pulled this quote from the Centers for Disease Control and Prevention (CDC) Lyme disease website for you to take a gander at:

> It is not uncommon for patients treated for Lyme disease with a recommended 2- to 4-week course of antibiotics to have lingering symptoms of fatigue, pain, or joint and muscle aches at the time they finish treatment. In a small percentage of cases, these symptoms can last for more than 6 months. Although sometimes called "chronic Lyme disease," this condition is properly known as "Post-treatment Lyme Disease Syndrome" (PTLDS). The exact cause of PTLDS is not yet known. Most medical experts believe that the lingering symptoms are the result of residual damage to tissues and the immune system that occurred during the infection. In contrast, some health care providers tell patients that these symptoms reflect persistent infection with *Borrelia burgdorferi* [Latin name for Lyme disease]. Recent animal studies have given rise to questions that require further research. Clinical studies are ongoing to determine the cause of PTLDS in humans (121).

To be honest, both viewpoints have validity. Individuals experience lingering symptoms due to both the persistence of the infection and residual damage. (Some of that residual damage is caused by the antibiotics themselves and by ill-equipped physicians ignorantly trying to treat Lyme.) But that's not the cause of Lyme disease, nor does the above explanation give you any information about what to do if you fall into that 90 percent of people. The bottom line remains the same: you still don't feel good.

As I've said, even though the name PTLDS is thought to be more accurate, I will use the term *chronic Lyme* from here on out because it's easier.

Simply said, chronic Lyme is really "Hey I got diagnosed with Lyme, I may or may not remember the initial infection, and it's been a long time since I've felt good."

How'd I Get Lyme in the First Place?

A tick, duh.

Although it's thought that most Lyme infections come from a deer tick bite, there are many additional carriers (known as vectors). These additional carriers include mosquitos, dog ticks, wood ticks, lone star ticks, rabbit ticks, and biting insects such as deer flies and horse flies. On top of that, common animals such as dogs, cats, horses, and birds also carry the disease. If you're pregnant, it can possibly be transmitted to your baby and cause a stillbirth (9). It's even thought to be an STD and transmitted through bodily fluids.

Now, although deer ticks are the only known transmitters of the disease, I would venture to guess that as research progresses, many of the animals and insects and other various methods of transmission will be shown to transfer the disease to humans, especially with the number of people who seem to have Lyme.

Simply said, most individuals probably have Lyme.

Wait a minute; you must explain that vast generalization. Most people have Lyme?

Yes, I believe most individuals have Lyme, but my goal is to show you by the end of this book that it doesn't matter whether you have Lyme, regardless of whether my statement is true or not. I reveal data on real Lyme individuals and explain our process of getting them better without ever killing their Lyme disease! My comments aren't meant to scare you - actually, quite the opposite. They're more to educate you about the unnecessary nature of your fear of Lyme and why it's not warranted in most cases. The bottom line is that if you use a proper and scientific testing approach, if you're trained to interpret and understand the test results, and if you're able to listen to what Lyme individuals are telling you, then a systematic, integrative, multifaceted treatment plan can get you better without having to kill Lyme disease.

But wait, you didn't completely answer the question: How did I get Lyme in the first place?

In my mind, there is not a question that many individuals have the disease yet are symptom free. Have you ever wondered why that is? Since I believe most individuals have Lyme, the better question is "Why am I experiencing symptoms of Lyme when many others do not?"

To allow entry and any subsequent development of Lyme symptoms, your immune system must have been compromised and/or your overall immune function must be deficient compared to those of healthy individuals. Individuals who are most susceptible to Lyme, its coinfections, and all their symptoms are individuals with poor immune function, especially when it comes to the persistence of symptoms. Moreover, healing Lyme is much more difficult if your immune system is suppressed. Most importantly, a healthy immune system is capable of clearing Lyme and a multitude of other pathogens and their resulting symptoms. This means if your immune system is healthy, you won't experience symptoms of the disease (11–16).

Simply said, the first condition for allowing entry and symptom development from Lyme and many other pathogens is a compromised immune system.

You may also wonder why some individuals who have Lyme experience few or no symptoms, while others endure numerous debilitating symptoms, causing their lives to become nearly impossible to navigate.

I'll dive into this, but first I must show you the possible causes for allowing entry and development of Lyme in the first place.

What Compromised My Immune System?

Proper healing requires proper questioning. I've already explained why you experience symptoms of Lyme in the first place: a compromised immune system. There are numerous other conditions Lyme seeks within its host – you - as it develops and causes symptoms, but regardless, something must have caused the initial disruption in your immune system.

At Lifestyle Healing Institute, we've spent many years researching the correlation among various causalities disturbing the integrity of multiple brain and bodily systems, including the immune system. In nearly all cases, when the immune system is compromised or imbalanced, it's not from the invading pathogen but through an external source. In other words, if you have symptoms from a pathogen such as Lyme, babesia, bartonella, and so on, your immune system must have been compromised at some point prior to your contracting said pathogen. Moreover, we show that poor immune function makes it difficult to treat Lyme. Now what are those causes?

I could go on and on about triggers for immune disturbances, but our research shows three major contributors. (Of course, there are more.) The most common and one of the most potent immune suppressants is stress and mental or emotional disturbances. To cause the amount of immune suppression seen with Lyme, the stress and/or disturbances must be chronic, which, to be honest, is not uncommon among Lyme individuals. Since most individuals affected by Lyme have some sort of stress, this definitely proves to play a major role in the initial disruption of the immune system.

The next cause of immune suppression and disruption is environmental/industrial toxins, which include fatty toxins (discussed in more detail in subsequent chapters) as well as drugs and pharmaceutical medications. These prove to be among the most potent and overlooked immune disruptors. Moreover, it's usually necessary to get you off drugs to ensure long-term healing and overall immune integrity. Our research and experience show that, even if stress is removed, it's still next to impossible to heal the immune system without addressing the medications you're on, as well as environmental/industrial toxicity. The last major immune disruptor is foods and food allergies. Everything is discussed in more detail in the final section of this book. In the end, immune suppression is most definitely multifactorial, as is everything.

Simply said, initial immune disruption is multifactorial, with environmental toxicity and medications playing a tremendous role.

The words detox and toxins (or environmental/industrial toxins) are used frequently in today's day and age, but these two words have different meanings depending on who you ask. Toxins tends to refer to cell waste, foreign materials, drugs, and more, while detox usually refers to getting rid of these toxins. I agree with these definitions; however, they usually don't encompass what I feel is one of the most common toxins we all encounter.

I want to simplify toxins into two types: fat soluble and water soluble. Water-soluble toxins (which dissolve in water) aren't as much of a concern, as they readily dissolve in water and are flushed out through urine. On the other hand, fat-soluble toxins (which dissolve in fats) don't dissolve easily in water and thus require additional measures for removal. When I'm talking about toxins, I am talking about cell waste, foreign materials, and so on, but I'm referring mainly to fat-soluble or fatty toxins (also referred to as environmental/industrial toxins) unless otherwise indicated. Not all toxins that pose threats are fatty, but the most common toxins that affect Lyme individuals tend to be fatty. When I'm talking about detox, I'm referring mainly to getting rid of fatty toxins.

There's been increasing emphasis on the role fatty toxins play in disrupting the brain and body, and even though there are mechanisms in the body that allow for excretion of fat-soluble toxins, it's estimated that 25 percent of the population has a genetic condition that makes this excretion extremely difficult. Some go as far as to say it's impossible to eradicate toxins with this genetic subset. This genetic condition is a subset of HLA-DRB-DBQ genetics (which I'll call the HLA gene) (17).

Although it's estimated that 25 percent of individuals have this genetic subset, more than 93 percent of our individuals possess the HLA gene. This comes as no surprise, as any disease, especially Lyme disease, is multifactorial. With the obvious suppression from stress, Lyme individuals are at high risk for fatty-toxin immune system suppression, which is something commonly seen in most chronic Lyme people who have the HLA gene.

Simply said, if you have Lyme, you probably have environmental toxicity. If you have Lyme, you also may have environmental-toxin susceptibility due to the HLA gene.

HLA-DRB-DBQ Genetics: What's That?

In the past ten years, there has been increasing research on susceptibility to fatty toxins. The medical field (mainly Dr. Shoemaker and his team) recently pinpointed the dramatic consequences to a subset of HLA-DRB-DBQ genetics (the HLA gene) regarding fatty toxins. There are many subsets of this gene, including the "dreaded gene," so labeled by Shoemaker; he says people with this subset don't respond well to treatment at all. Twelve years have elapsed, so I hope he's changed his thinking, because we've shown that's far from the truth. I have the dreaded gene; my dad has the dreaded gene. In fact, many of our Lyme individuals have the dreaded gene. However, our multifactorial approach initiates toxicity healing in a matter of weeks, even days, regardless of your genetic profile (and that includes methylation issues).

Anyway, what does susceptibility to fatty toxins mean?

People with this genetic subset cannot build antibodies to environmental/industrial toxins that are fat soluble. In other words, their bodies cannot locate and eliminate this type of toxin from their systems, resulting in massive storage of fatty toxins, which have alarming health consequences throughout the brain and body (17). Although there's an increased awareness of toxins, treatment for fatty/environmental toxicity isn't widely understood. (Don't worry—we get rid of them, and we'll prove it, too!)

What is the most common fatty/environmental toxin Lyme individuals should be aware of?

Mycotoxins.

Mycotoxins are toxins produced by numerous types of mold species. Mycotoxins cause what's known today as mold toxicity, and let me tell you: this can be quite alarming. If you still don't believe mold can cause significant health problems, check the year for me; it's the twenty-first century, right? Mycotoxins are extremely dangerous and well documented. In the brain, they can destroy the blood-brain barrier, the neurons (brain cells), and the ependymal cells (cerebrospinal fluid bordering cells). In the body, they can destroy the chondrocytes (cartilage cells) and cardiomyocytes (heart cells), inactivate DNA/RNA synthesis, and completely shut down our immunity, to name just a few disruptions (19–24). I go into the detrimental effects of mycotoxins in much more detail in section 4 if you are curious about more documented research.

I know many are skeptical of mold toxicity, but it can occur, and it can be quite damaging. Some argue airborne toxin exposure is unlikely, and our exposure is mainly from foods. I will show that both are possible, but airborne seems to be more damaging and more common. What I can tell you is that we make sure to test your home as part of our procedure to pinpoint where the toxicity is coming from, if there happens to be any. I can also say that we never hang our hat on one value from one system. One issue is never the cause of all your symptoms, and although mold can be damaging, it's not an exception. It plays a different role in each individual. I know some even argue about the validity of testing for mycotoxins in the first place, but when our individuals have positive values, their houses are also positive for mold. Moreover, the homes are remediated properly, and our treatment shows the removal of these toxins. Removal of these toxins is a necessary step, but not the only step, in achieving long-term healing. It's OK to be skeptical, but toxicity from mold should never be ignored, especially when it comes to Lyme and many other chronic diseases.

Other research points to various environmental toxins that are just as dangerous as mycotoxins; however, the most common and abundant toxins that individuals encounter are mycotoxins.

The National Institutes of Health (NIH) estimates that between 30 and 50 percent of homes have poor air quality due to mold (24). Studies show we spend up to 90 percent of our time indoors - hence, my emphasis on mold toxicity (18). If we were building fires indoors, I'd be talking about benzene. If we were painting our homes every other day, I'd be talking about toluene. The bottom line is we don't do these things; thus, the most common toxins Lyme individuals should be aware of are mycotoxins.

But it doesn't stop there, because coupled with the HLA gene, *all* fatty/environmental/industrial toxins are readily stored in the body, not just mycotoxins. This means that pesticides, food preservatives, industrial toxins, and many more pose a much greater threat to Lyme individuals than to the ordinary person.

So, do you still think you just have Lyme?

Simply said, if you have the HLA gene, you have a massive susceptibility to fatty toxins. Our research shows more than 93 percent of our individuals with Lyme have the HLA gene. Do you still think you have just Lyme?

With the HLA gene, not only are breathable toxins (like industrial toxins, pesticides, etc.) extremely dangerous, but the food you eat every day is suspect. There's an obvious debate about organic, non-GMO food versus conventional food, and I've probably used up my controversial comments for this book, so I'll save that argument for another day. However, what you can't argue with is documented research on the damage pesticides (environmental/industrial toxins) cause to your brain and body. To add to the insult, chronic Lyme individuals often have the HLA gene, which means consuming pesticides poses a much greater threat to them than to individuals without the HLA gene.

Anyway, I keep talking about fatty toxins, and some of you may wonder what they are.

What are some common fatty toxins?

- Environmental toxins: mold toxins (mycotoxins), both breathable and ingestible (breathable is worse)
- Industrial and environmental toxins: benzene and benzene derivatives, toluene, and more
- Industrial toxins: plastics, PVC, pesticides, preservatives

WHAT DOES ALL THIS MEAN?

People with the HLA gene can't build antibodies to fatty toxins and many environmental/industrial toxins, making it extremely difficult for them to eliminate these toxins from their systems. Toxins are readily stored, especially in areas that contain fat (fat cells, the brain, the myelin sheath, cell membranes) and begin to shut down the body's immune cells, including white blood cells, cytokines (immune signalers), and natural killer cells, almost immediately (19). This has alarming health consequences throughout an individual's brain and body. After the immune system begins to shut down from fatty toxins, it allows the free entry and development of infections such as Lyme disease, babesia, and bartonella, as well as other infectious pathogens.

Simply said, if you have Lyme, you probably have toxicity, whether environmental, industrial, or all of the above. If you have toxicity, your immune system is easily compromised and will not heal if you don't eliminate the toxins.

Why Do I Have Symptoms of Lyme?

This is the real question. Many diseases or infections don't affect every person every time. Have you ever wondered why? When it comes to Lyme disease and many other types of infection, the question is "Why do I have symptoms when others may not?"

If you've read the previous chapter, you should understand my view that many individuals carry Lyme disease. But even if you don't agree, you can't argue with the fact that there's a large disparity in the symptoms that individuals with Lyme experience.

First, a side note on another common disorder, and yes, as always, there is a point. Epstein-Barr virus is known to cause mononucleosis (mono). About 90 percent of adults have the Epstein-Barr virus, yet only about 25 percent of individuals actually get mono, which means only 25 percent of individuals experience symptoms from the virus (25).

The real question is "Why am I experiencing symptoms, but others are not?"

Mono proves to be merely a symptom of an underlying cause.

What is the most common underlying cause for experiencing symptoms from a pathogen?

A compromised immune system.

A compromised immune system not only allows entry and development of Lyme (and other pathogens) in the first place, but it's also the reason the pathogen is able to build a home (and then a fortress, a biofilm) to ultimately cause you to experience symptoms.

Many individuals who are infected with Lyme are also infected with bartonella, babesia, Epstein-Barr, mycoplasma, herpes, chlamydia, and many other infections. I have rarely, if ever, seen an individual with a Lyme infection and zero other accompanying infections. This vast number of overlapping pathogenic infections points to a much broader underlying cause beyond the individual infections. This overlap within Lyme individuals reveals the infections to be more like symptoms than causes. Through our research we've found these symptoms point toward immune dysfunction - a major amount of immune dysfunction. More importantly, after we restore the immune system, an individual can fight off infections at his or her own reasonable pace (if biofilm science is properly understood, which I talk about later). This causes individuals to shift toward that elusive majority, the majority who are not experiencing symptoms.

Simply said, a compromised immune system allows entry and development of Lyme symptoms and other common coinfections.

OK, so I'll just fix my immune system, and everything will be fine, right?

Not exactly.

That's a piece of the puzzle, but it runs much deeper than that. First off, something must have compromised your immune system in the first place. Even if you help heal the immune system so it's capable of fighting the symptoms of Lyme, you must ascertain why the infection happened in the first place. Otherwise, the solution will be only temporary; your immune system won't stay at a sufficient level to keep Lyme symptoms at bay. Adequate testing and questionnaires help determine answers for each individual, but if you remember, I've discussed the most common sources: stress and mental-emotional disturbances and toxicity, which includes drugs, and foods, and food allergies. Everything must be addressed to ensure your immune system functions adequately in the long term.

Now, after the causes that disrupted your immune system have been determined, you must understand there are also co-disruptions in other brain and bodily systems that must be considered to ensure proper healing. Ultimately, this is the reason a compromised immune system can account for the entry of Lyme and its initial symptom development; however, it cannot fully account for the debilitating Lyme symptoms. Moreover, it doesn't completely explain why the large majority of individuals with Lyme don't experience symptoms.

It's not enough to just remove the causes. You must heal the subsequent damages those causes have done to your brain and body; that's the key to true healing, and that's the true reason you're experiencing such debilitating symptoms. We've yet to see an individual who doesn't have co-disruptions. Here's a list of quantitative imbalances of brain and bodily systems we commonly encounter. (Obviously, this isn't everything.):

- Brain-chemistry imbalances
  - Excess excitatory neurotransmitters (electrifying brain chemicals)
  - Diminished inhibitory neurotransmitters (calming brain chemicals)
  - Underactive and overactive brain regions
  - Closed brain receptors
- Hormonal imbalances
  - Poor communication
  - Overall suppression
- Diminished gut integrity
  - Nutritional deficiencies
  - Poor absorption
  - Leaky gut syndrome
  - Imbalanced gut flora
  - Pathogens
- Poor blood flow and circulation
  - Dysregulations in osmolarity
  - Resistances to flow
  - Stagnate flow
  - Poor oxygen capacity and offloading
  - Lymphatic overload
- Mitochondrial dysfunction

And let's not forget two major aforementioned disruptions:

- Compromised immune system
  - Overactive autoimmunity
  - Suppressive autoimmunity
- Environmental/industrial toxicity

Not to mention the bevy of mental-emotional and mind-body issues every individual presents with. Once you master the art of healing each of the issues above, you must help individuals obtain a healthy mind and a healthy outlook of themselves and the world. Don't worry if you aren't familiar with many of the aforementioned issues, as I will explain them in Section 4.

Simply said, a compromised immune system is just one of many co-disruptions individuals with Lyme will experience.

I hope it's becoming clearer not only how but also why you have symptoms.

Lyme isn't the only thing that's causing these disruptions. As you will learn, any or all of the aforementioned issues can accurately - many times more accurately than Lyme - explain your symptoms, yet many people are quick to attribute all their symptoms solely to Lyme disease. That's just not the case - ever! Your Lyme symptoms always comes from multiple issues. Moreover, Lyme is usually not the underlying cause of your symptoms. More importantly, treating and removing conditions and disruptions to facilitate healing of your associated brain and bodily systems, without ever killing your Lyme, will get you better more than 90 percent of the time. Our research and approach show these issues are the true underlying causes of your symptoms.

As mentioned, multiple issues contribute to your disease state; therefore, everything must be addressed to ensure your best chance for healing. You can't just go and use nukes to kill Lyme at all costs. Not only are there consequences of this mentality, but it's also not a safe treatment approach by any means.

There is a process. There is a procedure. There is a method.

One of the most crucial aspects of understanding Lyme is understanding biofilms. Attacking Lyme or any of the 80 percent of infectious diseases that build biofilms requires complex science. If you truly understand the concepts behind biofilms and consider yourself a Lyme expert, then you must also be a coinfection expert, an environmental-toxicity expert, and a candida expert, because those issues and more are related to biofilms. Moreover, it's without question that opening biofilms and releasing the substances within them cause a detrimental change in brain chemistry, the immune system, blood flow, the GI system, and much, much more. These substances greatly affect individuals suffering from Lyme in as little as hours, if they decide to undergo Lyme treatment. This is commonly referred to as a Jarisch-Herxheimer reaction or die-off, which many attribute solely to killing Lyme; however, it's really from opening the floodgates of the biofilms. I discuss this subject in much more detail with documented research in section 2. I will show you why the definition of a Jarisch-Herxheimer reaction for biofilm-producing species isn't complete.

Simply said, Lyme is merely the façade of a bevy of other causes and disruptions often overlooked, misdiagnosed, and/or unaddressed. Understanding and healing disruptions and causes are ultimately what get you better.

Take a minute to reflect on this statement.

How Do I Determine Whether I Have Lyme?

For one thing, if you've experienced any of the co-disruptions I mentioned in the previous chapter, your probability of contracting Lyme and developing symptoms greatly increases. Many of these are common at one point or another, which is in part what led me to my conclusion that most individuals have Lyme. But hey, I'm an engineer, and engineers deal with concepts based in an objective nature.

So how do you test for Lyme?

Since Lyme is a stealth infection, it presents many problems for the testing process. The typical and most recognized tests aren't usually good enough to stand alone in diagnosing Lyme. Many of these accepted testing methods are based on antibody testing and are usually not as accurate as some of the more sophisticated testing that's available. The more sophisticated testing is typically not recognized by the FDA; therefore, it can't diagnose much of anything.

But wait - if you have Lyme, and Lyme is an infection, your body should produce antibodies to that infection. Why isn't this an accurate way of going about things?

The thought process is accurate, but it's just not that simple. First off, your immune system attacks different infections in different manners; thus, antibody testing may not be extensive enough to determine a Lyme infection. Another reason is there are more than one hundred identifiable strains of Lyme, and we're just beginning to understand the similarities and differences among them; it's not just a one-size-fits-all bug (26). On top of that, Lyme can exist in various forms: in its traditional spirochete but also in a cyst form, as well as an acellular membrane form (7). To make matters worse, to contract and develop Lyme symptoms, you must have been immunocompromised at some point; thus, your ability to produce adequate antibodies may not be strong enough to render a positive test.

Simply said, Lyme comes in many different strains, shapes, and sizes, making it difficult to diagnose and treat.

Besides Lyme itself being so sophisticated, here's a list of general reasons why antibody testing may not be the most accurate methodology. Remember, antibodies are one way your immune system recognizes and tries to eradicate invading pathogens:

- Antibodies may be present but not for that specific sample at that specific time (27).
- Antibodies don't necessarily indicate a current Lyme infection. (It could have been a prior infection from which you may or may not be experiencing symptoms.) (27).
- Lyme requires a multistep diagnosis involving numerous issues, not just antibody testing (27).
- There can be suboptimal precision in detecting some Lyme antibodies (27).
- Many medications lower antibody production (28).

There are many more reasons as well, but the three most common reasons among Lyme individuals are the lack of precision of Lyme testing, the fact that Lyme can hide within a biofilm, and the overall low immune function common among Lyme individuals. Oftentimes, these individuals will lack the ability to produce an adequate immune response in general, including adequate antibodies, to render a positive test.

I'll go through some tests and give you some take-home points for each one, but this is by no means meant to be a comprehensive and exhaustive list.

The most commonly encountered Lyme tests given at the first suspicion of Lyme are a western blot test, enzyme-linked immunosorbent assay (ELISA) testing, and a polymerase chain reaction (PCR). The first two tests are based on antibodies; thus, they have limitations for reasons I previously mentioned. I will say that if both your western blot and your ELISA tests come back positive, there is a high probability you have Lyme. Another note: there's much discussion concerning a positive p41 band on your western blot test; even without an overall positive test, if this band is positive, there's a high probability you have Lyme. Since more than 90 percent of the time, we do not need to kill your Lyme to heal your symptoms, I'm not concerned about the validity of the p41-band claims. The PCR test takes a sample of blood and basically replicates/expands your DNA numerous times; the results are then compared to other DNA sequencing (nucleotide sequencing). This comparison allows the clinician to determine whether there's a mutation in your DNA that indicates Lyme. The precision of this test is limited, and because there are so many strains and forms of Lyme, it's difficult to diagnose Lyme precisely with a PCR test.

These are probably the three most common tests you'll encounter (and yes, there are others), but I'd like to touch on some of the more precise tests available. Many are not FDA approved to diagnose Lyme; thus, interpretation is left to you and your physician, which is itself a limitation of these tests.

Companies like IgeneX, Fry Laboratories, and NeuroScience have more advanced tests that in many cases can be more accurate in diagnosing Lyme and its coinfections than traditional testing methods.

IgeneX has a good test for babesia; they run a fluorescence in situ hybridization (FISH) test, in which a blood sample is smeared, and babesia will light up if your blood has the infection. NeuroScience runs two pretty good tests for Lyme; they use specific immune-marker (cytokine and T/B lymphocyte) testing. This goes beyond antibody testing, as these markers are much more precise in showing the severity of your current immune response to Lyme. They can be paired with a western blot test to provide more accurate results. Probably the best test for Lyme, its coinfections, and pathogens seemingly unrelated to Lyme is from Fry Laboratories. Since everyone's blood has biofilms, a blood sample can be taken, and part of the biofilm can be illuminated. A fluorescent light specific to the DNA in biofilms is attached, making them light up and become more visible. This test shows any critter in your biofilm, and with experience, you can discern the severity of pathogenic biofilms. This test can be paired with a type of blood smear microscopic picture to analyze infections hiding inside or outside your cells, which also shows the integrity of the cells. Two limitations of the Fry Laboratories test are that it uses only one sample of blood and that biofilms are ubiquitous in nature, which sometimes leads to a false positive regarding what's considered a substantial number of biofilm critters. Since all these tests, including the Fry test, are expensive and usually not covered by insurance, repeat tests to ensure accurate diagnosis are difficult. On top of that, everyone has a degree of biofilm regardless of his or her current health status; thus, you must have an understanding of high bio-film exposure versus low biofilm exposure.

Other tests to note are a CD57, C3a and C4a protein test. CD57 is usually low in Lyme individuals, but it's also low in those with other disorders, including many chronic diseases and viral infections. It's a good quantitative marker to pair with symptoms demonstrating how chronically sick an individual is; however, its value isn't always an accurate indication of Lyme, because it jumps around quite a bit. C3a and C4a can be indicators of Lyme, but these tests must be run at a specific point because their quantities change depending on the progression of the disease. On top of that, C3a and C4a can be elevated in fatty toxin toxicity, which is much more common than Lyme.

I won't spend too much time discussing tests because you must run many of the tests simultaneously and then repeat them to ensure a precise diagnosis of Lyme disease. If you ask ten different doctors, you'll probably get nine different answers on the most accurate tests and methods for diagnosing Lyme, some of which merely use your past medical history and/or the process of elimination. This just shows how today's testing methods haven't caught up to some stealth infections like Lyme. Even then, you'll still be left with the same predicament: What do I do now?

An interesting point to note is the willingness of physicians to treat Lyme without a positive result. Because of the accepted stealth nature of the disease, many Lyme clinics will blindly treat the disease regardless of what the tests say. It may be one of the only diseases that have this trait. At times, this same blindness can be exhibited by the very individuals themselves. After such long-fought battles with the unknown, when a Lyme diagnosis is received, some stop their seemingly endless searches for the potential causes of their feeling the way they do. Many feel Lyme is the answer that makes the most sense, and I can understand that. However, in subsequent sections I will uncover much more accurate causalities that explain your symptoms much better than Lyme, regardless of a positive or negative Lyme test.

Simply said, there is no solid consensus on properly testing and diagnosing Lyme. Regardless, it doesn't matter whether you're positive; you don't have to treat Lyme to feel better.

Is Lyme Often Misdiagnosed?

If you've read the previous chapter, you now understand the limitations of current Lyme testing. These limitations lead us to an obvious question: Is Lyme often misdiagnosed? The short answer is yes. The long answer is still yes, but I'll explain a few details for you.

Quite simply, besides limitations in testing, the reason Lyme and various other diseases are often misdiagnosed is the landslide of symptoms that each individual presents. These symptoms, which are seen below, suggest diagnoses that many are familiar with.

The following is a list of a few diseases and symptoms that are often diagnosed in, seen in, and/or associated with people who have Lyme. This list is by no means meant to be exhaustive: Yersinia enterocolitica, Mycoplasma pneumoniae, Chlamydophila pneumoniae, Chlamydia trachomatis, Campylobacter jejuni, fatigue, headaches, lassitude, arthritis, dizziness, palpitations, dyspnea, chest pain, syncope, arthralgia, myalgia, CNS symptoms, paranoia, dementia, schizophrenia, bipolar disorder, panic attacks, major depression, anorexia nervosa, obsessive-compulsive disorder, depression, polyneuropathy, radiculopathy, skin lesions, erythema migrans, lymphadenopathy, heart disease, myocarditis, cardiomyopathy, pericarditis, eye-disease uveitis, conjunctivitis, optic neuritis, gastrointestinal complaints, urogenital symptoms, reactive arthritis, and Guillain-Barré syndrome (29–31).

Some are more common than others, and yes, there are many more. I could go to the trouble of listing them as well, but my point remains the same: Lyme is a stealth infection that resembles numerous other diseases, symptoms, and disorders. More importantly, you don't need to treat Lyme to feel better.

Simply said, yes, Lyme is easily and often misdiagnosed.

TWO

BIOFILMS

I was thinking about how to organize this next section, and I thought about using the same format as the first section to make it easier to follow, with questions such as "What are the symptoms?" However, I would be repeating myself, because the answers would remain the same. Lyme symptoms are the same as biofilm symptoms, as Lyme builds a biofilm. Biofilm symptoms are much worse because Lyme isn't the only thing that builds and hides within biofilms. As you'll discover while reading this section, there are numerous species and substances located within biofilms. When a biofilm is breached, these species and substances disrupt immune regulation, blood flow, brain chemistry, and hormones, and they're highly resistant and intricate and have been around for billions of years.

Thus, I decided to focus in this section on explaining the most current scientific research about biofilms to make it easy to understand. (Hopefully, I succeed in that task.) But the fact remains that biofilms are only one modality for treatment options you'll encounter when addressing individuals suffering from Lyme (or any biofilm disease). This doesn't understate their importance, but looking at one aspect will inherently leave you with a limited toolbox. When evaluating an individual, who's suffering from a chronic disease, especially Lyme disease, you must look at multiple modalities, not just Lyme and its biofilm. Hopefully, as you begin to delve into the bulk of information in this book, you'll understand more and more why this is true.

Now, let's get into some biofilms.

What Are Biofilms?
Biofilm: A Breeding Ground for Infections

In normal human terms, when speaking of infections, think of a biofilm as the fort or shield many pathogens build to survive in their host (you, in this case); this is the fortress I was referring to in the previous section. Remember, a pathogen is any entity that frequently causes infections in humans, such as bacteria, parasites, and viruses; Lyme is a pathogen, and so are babesia, bartonella, Rocky Mountain spotted fever, mycoplasma, HIV, and so on.

In more precise scientific terms, a biofilm is an extracellular matrix usually consisting of water, extracellular DNA, proteins, ions, and polysaccharides; **80 percent of infectious diseases will build one** within your body to increase their chances of survival. Yes, the overwhelming majority of all infections tend to build biofilms as their defense mechanism of choice. Biofilms form everywhere in nature, including in humans, where a free-flowing liquid passes by a smooth, solid surface (6, 7, 32). They are ubiquitous in nature.

A biofilm is a home for pathogens - a home where a pathogen can communicate with its friends and family, a home where everyone has a role, a home that provides food and shelter, a home that provides safety and promotes survival - just the same as your family, your friends, and your community, just the same as the roof over your own head.

Simply said, 80 percent of infectious diseases, including Lyme and many of its coinfections, build a biofilm. A biofilm is a fort or shield or a home pathogens build to promote their survival.

The term "biofilm" may be new to many of you, and that's OK - this whole section is about biofilms. But for chronic Lyme individuals, it's usually all too familiar. Lyme is part of that 80 percent of infectious diseases that build a biofilm (7).

I'll start off by giving you some examples of biofilms, and you'll be surprised how common some are. For example, a common but not widely known biofilm is dental plaque, one of the leading causes of tooth decay and gum disease. Water treatment facilities label biofilms as one of their most pesky issues. Biofilms are detected in almost every pipe that carries or drains fluids in your home as well as many facilities worldwide. Biofilms are involved in the extremely slippery rocks in rivers and creeks you're weary of while hiking. Biofilms form around medical devices such as catheters, pacemakers, and joint replacements (32, 33). There's evidence that many treatment-resistant and persistent chronic diseases have large biofilm components. For example, chronic cystic fibrosis is a biofilm disease. Persistent urinary tract, ear, and sinus infections have biofilm contributory factors. Biofilms also contribute to the formation of kidney stones. Atherosclerosis and endocarditis, both contributing to the number one cause of death in America, heart disease, have biofilm contributing components. Fungi (mold toxins, etc.) and candida species build biofilms. One of Lyme's most common coinfections, bartonella, builds a biofilm (32, 34-42); however, bartonella develops and persists only in immune-compromised individuals, just like Lyme disease (41). Hmm, I am sensing an underlying theme among these infections.

As usual, I could go on.

As Lyme begins to come to the forefront of the medical community, biofilms and biofilm research are of growing interest. But biofilms aren't a new concept at all. Biofilms are ubiquitous in nature as nearly 99.9 percent of bacteria would rather be stationary and form biofilms than be constantly moving in their free floating (planktonic) forms; biofilms are everywhere. Biofilms' strength is in numbers, especially when you go after them and stress them out. The earliest biofilms appeared on Earth about 4.5 billion years ago (32, 43)!

For those of you who don't know, the earth is about 4.54 billion years old (depending on whom you ask). And for you math wizards, that means that biofilms have been around for more than 99 percent of Earth's existence. On top of that, biofilms were around two billion years before their free floating (planktonic) counterparts (32). The earliest records of humans (although this is not fully agreed upon) date back, at most, two to three million years.

But enough of the history lesson; let's get back on topic.

Simply said, biofilms aren't a new concept. They've been around almost forever in terms of Earth's history. The earliest records of biofilms date back 4.5 billion years.

How Smart Are Biofilms?
Survival with the Least Resistance

In speaking about biofilms, I must explain two commonalities among all life on this planet. The first commonality is the pursuit of survival along the path of least resistance. In other words, in this case, if bacteria don't have to move, they won't; if they can be lazy, they will. Therefore, they will build biofilms because it's their path of least resistance (99.9 percent more likely, to be more precise). We humans aren't much different. Anyway, bacteria can go from their planktonic forms (common mobile, free-floating forms) to a sessile form (attached and clumped form - their biofilm form) (44).

"Why?" you ask.

Hey, why move if you don't have to?

Simply said, nearly all life on Earth wants to survive along a path of least resistance, and destructive pathogens are no exception. Biofilms are their survival tactic, their path of least resistance.

Biofilms' Intricate Design and Communication System

Bacteria's sessile (biofilm) form not only makes it easier for them to exist but also makes them much more efficient. Numerous studies show biofilm producing species have their own networks designed for survival. They have their own nutrient, oxygen saturation, and metabolic systems. They have roads like a city, shipping in nutrients and removing waste. They can even switch back to their free-floating forms if they so please. If supplies run low, they roll or detach to invade other tissues and gather up the nutrients they desire. They also have an extremely intricate communication system known as quorum sensing; in other words, they talk to one another. Current research shows biofilm producing species designate a whopping 10 percent of their genetic code to this communication system. They have signaling cells and target cells whose activities are highly coordinated and integrated (43–46).

Moreover, biofilm species usually operate under the principle that there is strength in numbers. Bacteria tend to congregate together with multiple biofilm producing species. The more species, the more resistant the biofilm becomes (32, 43). In other terms, a biofilm with only Lyme disease is less difficult to penetrate than a biofilm with Lyme and common coinfections, such as bartonella or candida overgrowth. If your body were a country, a biofilm would be a city - an extremely diverse, large, integrated, role specific community that varies in size but is inherently inevitable in any body or any country. **Simply said, a biofilm is melting pot of diverse, smart, coordinated, and integrated pathogenic species that function as a large, urban city.**

Biofilms are simpler than cities because in the end they're just homes for pathogens, homes that exist in a city or out in the country. Pathogens would rather exist in cities, but in the end, they just want a community and a roof over their heads. Think about it: Would you rather live life zipping around on roads and highways, left to fend for your own food, your own nutrients, by yourself (the free-floating form)? Or would you rather live in a nice cozy home with all your friends and family surrounding you in a self-sustaining community (the biofilm form)? I already know the answer to my rhetorical question, considering most, if not all, of us would have chosen the latter.

We'd rather have divisible roles; support systems; and most importantly, safety. Safety ensures survival, and a pathogen's biofilm provides that safety; it provides pathogens with longevity that promotes survival within a sophisticated network. We humans have similar systems and methods of survival. We, too, have nutrients, oxygen saturation, and metabolic systems. We, too, have an intricate communication system, albeit using neurotransmitters, hormones, and much more. We, too, have strength in numbers. We, too, want a role specific multi-contributory community. We, too, want to be safe.

I wonder how all that came about.

But we're much smarter; we have nice, large brains.

I digress…

Simply said, biofilm producing species would rather exist in an attached biofilm form as opposed to free-floating, as it's much more efficient for survival being in a self-sustaining, intricate system known as a biofilm.

Where Do Biofilms Tend to Grow?

This bacterial biofilm growth occurs in numerous places in the body but tends to find itself in the largest number, causing the most detriment, in the gut as well as the bloodstream. Remember, biofilms form where there's a flowing liquid next to a smooth, solid surface, such as the circulatory system, with the blood (liquid) and walls of the blood vessels (smooth and solid), and the GI system, with the mucus/water (liquid) and the GI tract (smooth and solid). Biofilms are found in the brain and nervous tissue as well (7).

As biofilm growth builds, the blood begins to aggregate and becomes more viscous (thicker - honey is more viscous than water), making transport difficult. It comes as no surprise that increases in biofilm production lead to an increase in clotting factors (fibrinogen, platelets, etc.), thus leading to symptoms such as high blood pressure, constipation, chronic migraines, overall increases in electrical activity in the brain, and much more.

When blood transport is disrupted, everything is disrupted. Tissues, including the brain, can't get the proper nutrient delivery or expunge their waste, which leads to a bevy of health issues. This is the reason why blood transport is so crucial in treating any disorder, especially chronic disease, and Lyme is no exception.

Simply said, a biofilm provides a platform where Lyme and other infectious diseases have a safe haven to hang out, gather nutrients, and communicate in their cozy forts in your body.

Biofilms are pretty crazy, huh? They are super intricate, having evolved and mastered their techniques for billions of years.

But wait, there's more.

Survival at All Costs: Biofilm Resistance

I've already discussed the intricate communication and metabolic systems all biofilms inherently possess, but as mentioned, biofilms run much deeper than that. If you've been keeping track, you may be wondering about the second commonality among all life on this planet. I haven't told you yet, but I'm about to now. Maybe that's poor organization, considering all the information listed between now and then, or maybe I did it on purpose because that information was pretty cool and interesting, wasn't it? Anyway, to remind you, the first commonality among all life on this planet is the pursuit of survival along a path of least resistance.

The second commonality among all life on this planet is that nothing wants to die. And if life is forced to die, it'll do everything in its power to make its death meaningful by making one final statement.

When it comes to biofilm producing species, this trait manifests in resistance. This resistance is most commonly seen through three phenomena:

1. Biofilms' protection from your own immune system
2. Biofilms' response to antibiotic use
3. Biofilms' final Jarisch-Herxheimer reaction (biofilm species' final statement)

Biofilms' Protection from Your Own Immune System

At the beginning of this book, I discussed two types of invasive pathogens. When your body is under attack from any pathogen, your immune system tries to defend your brain and body and get rid of the invader. To simplify the overall mechanism, your body has monitoring cells, tagging cells, signaling cells, killing cells, and more. Most are designed, in the end, to tell your killer cells to go after foreign invaders. One of your main killing cells is macrophages, which literally engulf and eat these foreign invaders. This intricate communication and defense system is designed not only to kill foreign invaders but also to ensure your body doesn't mistake your own cells, your own tissues, with these foreign invaders. (The latter is what goes wrong in autoimmunity.)

This process works for one type of invasive pathogen, and for most infections, this mechanism is extremely effective. However, for the other type of invasive pathogen, which is what this book's all about, this mechanism isn't effective. It's not effective because this type of pathogen builds biofilms. Biofilms are nearly completely shielded from your immune system (hence, my use of the word *fortress* to describe them) (47). That means the previous paragraph is largely irrelevant when it comes to biofilm producing pathogens, including Lyme and many of its coinfections. This is the first way that biofilm producing species are resistant; biofilm producing species are largely shielded from your immune system.

Let me repeat, Lyme is largely shielded from your immune system.

But again, it runs deeper than that.

In fact, your body still tries to attack these species within their biofilms and send killer cells (macrophages) to eat them (phagocytosis) (47). But their efforts are futile, as some of your macrophages actually die in their attempts to kill bugs within the biofilm. Your immune system simply can't kill species with any effectiveness whatsoever if they're encased within biofilms.

Simply said, the second commonality among life on this planet is that nothing really wants to die. In accordance with this trait, many pathogens, like Lyme, build biofilms to ensure their survival. Biofilm producing species like Lyme are almost completely shielded from your immune system.

Biofilms' Response to Antibiotic Use

Now let's get to the second way that biofilm producing species are resistant: their resistance to the use of antibiotics.

If you remember the history lesson in the first section, you understand when and how Lyme was discovered. The point of that section was to show the time period in which Lyme was discovered, which dictated the use of antibiotics in its treatment. Many allopathic doctors are still trained with the mentality "bacterial infection = antibiotics." There's just one problem: Lyme (after two weeks of initial infection) finds its way to its friends and joins and contributes to biofilms. This renders antibiotics completely ineffective in eradicating chronic Lyme disease and every biofilm producing species, for that matter.

Not only are antibiotics completely ineffective in eradicating chronic Lyme disease, but they actually cause much brain and body damage. I'll discuss the damage later on and here discuss how resistant biofilm species are to antibiotics.

I get pushback every time I talk about the ineffectiveness of antibiotics in the treatment of Lyme disease and other biofilm producing chronic diseases. To be honest, I just don't get it. Not only have we shown it through the treatment of individuals suffering from chronic Lyme at our facility, but the large majority of research also demonstrates this to be true. Because of the inherent pushback I may get from my opinions in this book, I've decided it's best to include some of the quantitative research I've done that led me to this conclusion, and you can read it for yourself.

Antibiotics are completely ineffective at eradicating any biofilm producing infection, including chronic Lyme. Let me repeat that.

Antibiotics are completely ineffective at eradicating any biofilm-producing infection, including chronic Lyme.

Here's the research:

Direct observations have clearly shown that biofilm bacteria predominate, numerically and metabolically, in virtually all nutrient-sufficient ecosystems. Therefore, these sessile [biofilm] organisms predominate in most of the environmental, industrial, and medical problems and processes of interest to microbiologists. If biofilm bacteria were simply planktonic cells that had adhered to a surface, this revelation would be unimportant, but they are demonstrably and profoundly different. **We first noted that biofilm cells are at least 500 times more resistant to antibacterial agents [antibiotics].** (48)

Formation of biofilm communities turned out to be one of the main survival strategies of bacteria in their ecological niche. **Bacteria in attached condition in biofilm are protected from the environmental damaging factors and effects of antibacterial substances [antibiotics] in the environment and host organism during infection.** (49)

Biofilms have been shown to be pathogenetic factors responsible for chronization of infectious process. The data are presented illustrating ubiquitous nature of biofilms, their structural and functional characteristics, and modern methods for the study of microbial communities. **The discussion is focused on the role of biofilms in chronization of infectious process, enhanced resistance of biofilm organisms to antibiotics and its underlying mechanisms.** (50)

Bacteria survive in nature by forming biofilms on surfaces and probably most, if not all, bacteria (and fungi) are capable of forming biofilms. A biofilm is a structured consortium of bacteria embedded in a self-produced polymer matrix consisting of polysaccharide, protein and extracellular DNA. Bacterial biofilms are resistant to antibiotics, disinfectant chemicals and to phagocytosis [macrophages' way of killing invading pathogens] and other components of the innate and adaptive inflammatory defense system of the body. It is known, for example, that persistence of staphylococcal infections related to foreign bodies is due to biofilm formation. Likewise, chronic *Pseudomonas aeruginosa* lung infections in cystic fibrosis patients are caused by biofilm growing mucoid strains. (51)

Many bacteria grow on surfaces forming biofilms but often high dosages of antibiotics cannot clear infectious biofilms. (52)

Many bacteria can form aggregates on interfaces, called biofilms, where they are much more protected against toxic agents such as antibiotics or antibodies. (53)

Excessive and indiscriminate use of antibiotics to treat bacterial infections has led to the emergence of multiple drug resistant strains. (54)

It has been discovered that bacteria present within the QS-mediated biofilm are up to 1,000 times more resistant to antibiotics than the planktonic [free-floating] forms...The myth—Antibiotics inhibit the growth of the microbes and may eventually kill it. (46)

Bacteria can switch between planktonic forms (single cells) and biofilms, i.e., bacterial communities growing on solid surfaces and embedded in a matrix of extracellular polymeric substance. **Biofilm formation by pathogenic bacteria often results in lower susceptibility to antibiotic treatments and in the development of chronic infections.** (55)

Bacterial biofilms are highly recalcitrant to antibiotic treatment, which holds serious consequences for therapy of infections that involve biofilms... Induced resistance factors include those resulting from induction by the antimicrobial agent itself [the antibiotic]. Biofilm antibiotic resistance is likely manifested as an intricate mixture of innate and induced mechanisms. **Many researchers are currently trying to overcome this extreme biofilm antibiotic resistance.** (56)

Formation of these sessile [biofilm] communities and their inherent resistance to antimicrobial agents [antibiotics] are at the root of many persistent and chronic bacterial infections. (57)

Bacterial populations produce a small number of dormant persister cells that exhibit multidrug tolerance. **All resistance mechanisms do essentially the same thing: prevent the antibiotic from hitting a target.** (58)

Biofilms are resistant to antibiotics, disinfectives and phagocytosis [macrophages' mechanism for killing invader cells]. (59)

But hey, let's use antibiotics; they seem to work well. They definitely have science on their side. If I could use emojis in this book, I'd throw up a sarcastic smiley face and a thumbs-up.

I could go on - and quite honestly, sometimes I want to, out of principle - but I'll contain myself.

Let's check in and see what my man Albert Einstein said about that mentality: "Insanity: doing the same thing over and over again and expecting different results."

But seriously, do you understand antibiotic treatments will fail nearly every time when treating biofilm producing diseases like chronic Lyme?

Simply said, antibiotics will fail almost every time when it comes to treating chronic Lyme disease.

Wait, what?

Antibiotics will fail almost every time when it comes to treating chronic Lyme disease.

The persistence of Lyme symptoms is due to the fact that many physicians are incapable of changing their views, of reading the latest research. Much of the persistence of Lyme symptoms stems from the very way we are accustomed to treating the disease. This persistence of symptoms in and of itself proves we need another way.

Are you beginning to understand why so many individuals suffer from the debilitating symptoms of chronic Lyme?

Do you understand the need for a different viewpoint, a different way to heal Lyme?

So, as you're sitting there getting an IV of multiple potent antibiotics, after ingesting even more, now you know this isn't the best way to treat Lyme - at all. Actually, it has little to no scientific backing whatsoever. (See above!)

As I've said numerous times, this book is written for you, the individual suffering from Lyme, to provide you with some education, some answers, and another way - a better way.

I want you to remember to ask yourself "Is my doctor even capable of treating my Lyme disease?"

If he or she is using antibiotics for your chronic Lyme, the answer is surely no.

More importantly, if your doctor wants primarily to use antibiotics in your treatment of Lyme disease, then he or she isn't experienced in healing the disease. Your doctor isn't using an efficient, scientific, nondamaging, non-time-consuming treatment approach.

Honestly, how frustrated would you be if you were a researcher from any of the articles cited above?

Obviously, the information and the science exist, as I found those articles within thirty minutes (not an exaggeration). I love researchers; I wanted to be a researcher and developer, which is why I went to school for chemical engineering. I wanted to design drugs. I even told my mom when I was sixteen years old, early in my junior year of high school, "I'm going to be a chemical engineer and design drugs. I don't understand why they spend billions of dollars on AIDS research, and no one can fix it. If you gave me a billion dollars and a seemingly unlimited amount of time, I could figure out AIDS." Good thing my mom loves me, because as you can see, I've been annoyed at the inadequacies of the implementation of research since I was sixteen. Ironically enough, I now specialize in developing programs to detox people off medications - funny how things work out.

But as a sixteen-year-old, I was ignorant to the inherent laziness of the human population - more specifically, the medical community. Hey, why move if you don't have to? Why change if you don't have to? I'm not going to group everyone in this category, as there are some brilliant physicians and individuals out there who put in the necessary work to help people suffering from chronic disease. (I presently work with one.) But the truth is most do not. I wish it weren't true, but it is. As I've stated, I feel your initial physician could have stopped the progression of your symptoms into the debilitating burden they are now. The blame for your progression is given to Lyme when in reality your physicians have failed you; the medical community has failed you.

As I progressed through college, I realized how, but more importantly why, physicians were failing individuals on an alarming level. The research needed to make a change existed, yet nothing was happening. "Why?" I asked myself. Besides obvious restrictions like politics and money (which are immense hurdles), I've concluded that one of the main reasons is that the interpreters of this information, the physicians, don't like to read or do much research at all. (And if they do, it's usually from one source.) They're often stubborn and don't like being told what to do; I can understand that.

Since they don't read, they have stopped interpreting data that is being published by knowledgeable and respectable scientists and researchers worldwide. Or since they don't understand the information, they arrogantly toss it aside as if it was nonsense. "What physicians aren't up on, there're down on," it's been said - hence, my career shift. Hey, I'll read; it's not that difficult. And I must add I have the benefit of seeing the transformation of our individuals based on my interpretations, which led to important adjustments not only to their treatment protocols but to my own fundamental conceptualization of healing.

Reading, interpreting, and enacting adjustments as needed reinforced my philosophy: let your body be your best defense system. Let your body be your most efficient and sophisticated healing tool. Our bodies don't want to die either, so let them do what they're designed to do: survive. If we keep trying to come up with sophisticated solutions to wipe out bacteria, they'll use their innate abilities to survive and leave us continually searching for new mechanisms to kill them.

Simply said, there is research showing how ineffective antibiotics are in treating many chronic diseases, including chronic Lyme, yet this information is often ignored. Let your body be your best defense system, your most efficient and sophisticated healing tool. Our bodies don't want to die either, so let them do what they're designed to do: survive.

Now, if bacteria were resistant just to antibiotics, it might not be that bad. But that's not the case. When you provoke biofilms with an antibiotic attack, they respond. Biofilms and the species within them are much savvier than many realize. As explained previously, when under attack, pathogens do whatever it takes to survive, which includes elaborate survival adaptations. This isn't uncommon for pathogens and bacteria, but what exactly is the result of these adaptations? The most common adaptation is that the biofilm becomes more resistant not only to the strain of antibiotics used but also to any subsequent treatment, whether antibiotic or not (60, 61).

It's even more interesting to note that studies have shown that these species become more resistant by various mechanisms, but I found this next study quite interesting, and it also further supports my philosophy.

The study shows that when Escherichia coli (E. coli), one of the most researched bacteria and a biofilm producing bacteria, was treated with antibiotics, two distinct adaptations occurred. What's even more interesting is researchers used the same stimulus and the same antibiotics and noted two distinct adaptations. This indicates resistance to our attacks is probably encoded within the bacteria's genetic code (61).

The first mutation was the most common; the bacteria simply became more resistant. However, the other was much more intriguing and frightening. The pathogen mutated by stealing a piece of DNA from a leftover virus. The same stimulus (antibiotics) led to two distinct adaptations, both of which prolonged survival and increased resistance to any subsequent treatment (61).

Antibiotics give us a false sense of security, and our indiscriminate use of them has led to adaptive resistance.

Simply said, biofilm species, including Lyme, become more resistant from the use of antibiotics. This resistance is seen in multiple, complex ways depending on the species within the biofilm.

In fact, this massive biofilm resistance to antibiotics has led to research into and the use of biofilm communication disrupters, known as quorum-sensing inhibitors (QSIs). Remember, quorum sensing is the way biofilm species communicate. Biofilms have an intricate communication system known as quorum sensing, to which 10 percent of their genetic code is dedicated. Logic led us to the idea that we should disrupt the communication, thus stopping the biofilm's growth and progression. It surely seemed logical. There's only one thing wrong: biofilm bacteria have been around for 4.5 billion years. Predictably, the tested bacteria adapted to the QSIs and became resistant to them also (46). Many are advocates for natural medicine, as I am, so you may already be against antibiotics and understand the drawbacks of using them. You may be thinking, "Yeah, but what about natural medicine studies on biofilm producing species?" Many QSIs are natural herbs and substances, and many are plant derived (84).

Although I am heavily biased toward natural medicine, this isn't a question of being naturally or pharmaceutically based. This philosophy is rooted in the nature of biofilms themselves, not the tools used. Many value the use of herbs or nutraceuticals to boost immunity in the treatment of Lyme disease. Numerous herbs can break biofilms; some natural derivatives even "trick" biofilms into opening their channels to further enhance the effectiveness of eliminating Lyme. Oftentimes, physicians and individuals use enzymes to dissolve biofilms. Some argue many immune-modulating herbs are adaptogenic: they increase resistance to the adverse effects of long-term stress. Many speak of the potency of liposomal herbs and vitamins. All these treatments are great, but not for Lyme and not for many biofilm producing species. When it comes to Lyme specifically, it's unnecessary more than 90 percent of the time. I'm sorry, but it's the truth.

An understanding of immune function is crucial, but contrary to what many believe, you don't need to use any immune modulators to restore immune function. If you truly understand immune function, you know that immune modulation occurs naturally in the great majority of individuals if the underlying causes are addressed. More than 80 percent of our individuals achieve nearly complete immune function restoration in a matter of weeks without ever using immune adaptogens, enhancers, or modulators. Please note this has nothing to do with the effectiveness of natural medicine versus allopathic (mainstream) medicine. This has nothing to do with herbs versus pharmaceuticals. This has to do with the nature of biofilms themselves;

we've been underestimating their intelligence and innate ability to survive for thousands of years. It's time to wake up and address this problem from a completely different angle. Whether attacked by natural or synthetic means (like antibiotics), biofilms adapt; this reaction is part of their foundation. But hey, let's keep trying to kill them; let's keep trying to kill Lyme.

Simply said, not only are antibiotics ineffective at eradicating Lyme, but antibiotics make biofilm species (Lyme included) much more resistant to any subsequent therapy. Contrary to what many believe, this isn't a question of natural versus synthetic, herbs versus antibiotics; all therapies underestimate the innate intelligence of biofilms. The resistance and intricacies of biofilms are what dictate the need for another way.

Does Lyme Exist in Biofilms Solely as a Traditional Spirochete?

I want to show you how smart and intricate a biofilm system and the species that lie within truly are, because this is one of the main reasons you shouldn't kill Lyme. Therefore, I want to spend a brief chapter discussing the fact that Lyme doesn't exist solely as the well-known spirochete to further emphasize the intricate nature of these species. As I've mentioned, the latest tests involve examining biofilms and the organisms located within them, similar to a Fry test, which was discussed at the end of Section 1. These analyses show pathogens like Lyme and their ability to assume multiple different forms and appearances. Lyme exists in the following forms (and probably many more):

1) Traditional spirochete form (7)
2) Cystic form (7)
3) Acellular cell membrane form (Without a cell membrane, which is the gatekeeper of the cell, it is cell wall deficient.) (7)

As mentioned, most individuals with Lyme know about the traditional spirochete shape, but as Lyme builds a biofilm and is attacked by substances such as antibiotics, it responds by changing its form, usually into the cystic form. More research is needed to determine whether each form has the same properties as the traditional spirochete (I'd guess they have different properties), but these multiple forms have been proven to exist. This shows how intricate Lyme, its biofilm, and its adaptations can truly be. It shows why you need a truly innovative approach that looks at multiple modalities, including not only Lyme itself but also the resulting years of damage to your brain and body.

Lyme and Its Coinfections

When I started writing this book, I tried to determine a solid outline that adequately explained my research as well as my take on Lyme disease. It's hard for me because I could write an entire book on many of these topics, yet most, if not all, must be mentioned and discussed in some capacity regarding Lyme. All of them have a role; however, some topics inherently take a back seat, and I can't spend as much time as I'd like to fully shed light on all the topics. This doesn't mean they're any less important. However, I wanted to write at least one chapter on Lyme and its coinfections. Not only are they important, but they also emphasize my philosophy on Lyme. There are numerous coinfections - far too many to list - but I'll discuss three of them, albeit briefly: babesia, bartonella, and mycoplasma. They're different in nature but also similar, in that they tend to cause symptoms because of a compromised immune system.

Simply said, bartonella, babesia, and mycoplasma are three of the most common coinfections seen in Lyme patients and develop in the same fashion: through a compromised immune system.

Babesia, bartonella, and mycoplasma often begin with a high fever and chills, as do many infections. In terms of biology and biochemistry, cooling tends to slow and/or stop, and heating tends to speed up, sometimes to the point of degradation. Thus, it makes sense that many invading pathogens elicit this response, as excessive heat may be our bodies' attempt to degrade (and hopefully kill) the invading pathogen. Most of the time, individuals with Lyme or any of its coinfections don't remember initially contracting the infections. As 90 percent of Lyme individuals don't remember getting the bull's-eye rash, many also don't remember their initial fevers either. The main reason many individuals don't recall the initial infection is that their immune systems were vastly compromised, thus allowing infections to enter and develop in the first place; they were actually so compromised (so autoimmune) that the infection didn't elicit an immune response at all. That's why many don't remember getting the bite, seeing the bull's-eye, getting a fever, or even being sick at all at the time of the initial infection.

Simply said, the main reason you contract infections and develop symptoms in the first place (compromised immunity) is the same reason the vast majority of individuals don't remember getting sick at the time of the initial infection.

Babesia was initially discovered way back in the late 1800s but has been referenced as early as Ramses II around 1250 BC. You can think of babesia as being similar to malaria, although not as deadly. Malaria is one of the deadliest killers in the world, with 438,000 deaths and a reported 214 million cases in 2015 (63, 64). Babesia crawls into the red blood cells, which carry oxygen, and inflames them. Red blood cells are about eight microns (0.000008 meters) wide, and some of your body's blood vessels (one of the fundamental components of your body's main fluid transport system) are as small as three microns. Cells inflamed with an infection like babesia are larger and have more difficulty moving through your body's transport system. This also increases inflammation throughout the brain and body. Think about putting a golf ball into a cup. Now imagine putting a basketball in that same cup; it would be quite difficult. This is an extreme example, but you get the point. This is what babesia and other similar intracellular infections can inflict. Not only does this contribute to overall systemic inflammation, but it disrupts blood flow, oxygen transport and delivery, and more. Oftentimes intracellular infections cause enlarged red blood cells (increased RDWs) as well as low iron and nutritional blood values (hemoglobin, ferritin, MCV, MCH, MCHC, and more). Sometimes they result in low red blood cell count in general, due to the spleen destroying the abnormal, inflamed cells. It's not surprising that individuals with babesia experience high blood pressure; heart arrhythmia; headaches; migraines; and in some cases, neurological symptoms, in addition to many other common symptoms (62, 63). Although Lyme disease is pushed to the forefront, babesia, along with bartonella and mycoplasma, is truly more of a concern than Lyme.

While babesia is located mainly inside red blood cells (it is intracellular), bartonella is located mainly outside the cells (it is extracellular). Its initial discovery is credited to A. L. Barton in 1909, and it's now known that bartonella functions mainly as an opportunistic pathogen. In simpler terms, bartonella is much more likely to cause detrimental effects in individuals with compromised immune systems. No surprise there, as this is also true of Lyme, babesia, and numerous other pathogens. As with babesia, many symptoms of bartonella resemble those of Lyme, making it difficult to diagnose accurately. However, if a live blood analysis, a dark film test, or any high-powered microscopic red blood cell–testing method is employed, bartonella and babesia can be illuminated.

One symptom that's unique to bartonella is the appearance of red, streaky stretch marks on the hips, shoulders, back, and more. Both babesia and bartonella are mainly red blood cell infections. Since the life-span of red blood cells is about 120 days, "experienced" physicians will administer antibiotic therapy for about five months or more!

What many fail to understand is that these species are extremely savvy. Bartonella has an innate ability to adapt rapidly to changing environments, making survival easier inside its hosts. It is also evasive of many antibiotics. It has two outer shields to prevent antibiotic entry (two cell walls), enzymes that can degrade antibiotics (beta-lactamases), and pumps that can rapidly rid it of antibiotics (efflux pumps). Oh, and that's in addition to its inherent ability to build and live within biofilms.

Simply said, the symptoms of bartonella and babesia resemble those of Lyme; however, bartonella and babesia often affect red blood cells (cells that carry oxygen) and can be seen without surrounding biofilms. This makes both of them more dangerous than Lyme in numerous ways.

The last pathogen I'd like to talk about is mycoplasma. Mycoplasma is much smaller than anything I've discussed thus far, and it's another common and often-overlooked coinfection of Lyme disease. Mycoplasma is super tiny; if we see bartonella as microscopic, bartonella sees mycoplasma as microscopic. About twelve bartonella bacteria can fit inside one of your red blood cells, while about four thousand mycoplasma bacteria can fit inside your cell. Remember, your red blood cells are about eight one-millionths of a meter in diameter. As I said, mycoplasma is super tiny.

How can it exist in such a microscope form?

It basically sheds the most common type of machinery bacteria have: a cell wall, the shield surrounding the epicenter of most bacteria. This allows it to reproduce and move quickly throughout the body. Mycoplasma bacteria prove to be resistant to antibiotic therapy. Surprise, surprise. They also prove to be very resistant to common pasteurization techniques and have been tested to persist in more than half of all dairy products. There are numerous strains revealed that affect many different parts of the body. The Fry test detects mycoplasma and other coinfections in your biofilm. The most common coinfections are protozoa and coccobacilli, such as chlamydia, which is an STD also carried by ticks that carry Lyme. As with Lyme, most individuals probably have some sort of mycoplasma bacteria, especially considering mycoplasma's ability to replicate and survive.

Again, reiterating one of the major themes of this book, who exhibits symptoms of mycoplasma infections (and pretty much every infection)? Individuals with compromised immune function.

Are you sensing the theme by now? I surely hope so. This is also true with Lyme, bartonella, babesia, and the large majority of infections. Actually, these species often select hosts with immune malfunction to promote their own survival, and honestly, this isn't a new concept. What is a new concept is that symptoms associated with Lyme are usually not a result of Lyme. This is often true with Lyme coinfections as well.

Biofilms' Final Jarisch-Herxheimer Reaction

As with biofilms, a Herxheimer reaction is another term that chronic Lyme individuals are all too familiar with. It is most commonly referred to as a die-off or a Herx among Lyme individuals and more accurately known as the Jarisch-Herxheimer reaction (JHRxn). The discovery of this effect is credited to two individuals: Adolf Jarisch, who first noted it way back in 1895, and Karl Herxheimer, who confirmed it in the early 1900s. This effect was first noted in the fifteenth century. Jarisch and Herxheimer discovered the effect, noting the reactions of individuals after being treated for syphilis, which has similarities to Lyme. Jarisch proposed that the reaction (most commonly seen as fevers, chills, blood pressure changes, heart rate changes, skin reactions, anxiety, and more) was caused by toxins being released from inside the spirochete of syphilis (65, 66).

As I stated earlier, nothing wants to die, and if they must die, pathogens do everything they can to make one last statement to make their deaths meaningful. This last-ditch effort is a JHRxn. Fast-forward to today, and it's most commonly seen when trying to kill Lyme disease and many other biofilm-producing species. Basically, when you threaten the survival of pathogens, they respond by releasing toxins. These toxins get released into your gut, your bloodstream, your brain, and anywhere else where there's a biofilm. The toxins then make their way to every part of your body, often through the bloodstream. Jarisch-Herxheimer reactions cause increases in, among other substances, tumor necrosis factor alpha (TNF-alpha) and matrix metallopeptidase 9 (MMP-9), which initiate immune reactions in both the brain and body hopefully to clear out toxins (17). If treatment is overdone, as it usually is with many Lyme therapies, your own cells and tissues are attacked as well. Elevations in TNF-alpha and MMP-9 are enough by themselves to make you feel terrible, but in excess, they cause your immune system to attack you as well, further contributing to the autoimmunity commonly seen among Lyme individuals. Sometimes the effects of a Jarisch-Herxheimer reaction can be felt for days, weeks, months, or even years after treatment has ended, because the massive increase in immune signaling remains for a long time. This leads individuals to feel as though they're in a constant state of die-off, even if they're no longer receiving treatment. Regardless of their initial locations, toxins make their way to various other brain and bodily systems via your bloodstream. Your brain and body respond the same way they would to any toxin (which I'll show you through our own research in Section 4):

- Increased electrical activity in the brain
- Compromised blood flow
- Increased inflammation
- Disruptions in immunity/autoimmunity
- Increased pathogenic exposure
- Increased environmental/industrial toxin exposure
- Increased liver stress
- Disruptions in the GI system
- Hormonal disturbances

This also leads to an exacerbation of any symptoms you're currently experiencing. Many individuals even develop additional symptoms they weren't experiencing prior to attacking Lyme! Here are just a few of the most commonly experienced symptoms:

- Brain fog
- Decreased cognition and memory
- Anxiety
- Sleep issues
- Increased pain
- Fevers
- Chills
- Fatigue
- Vomiting
- GI distress
- Headaches/migraines
- Changes in blood pressure
- Changes in heart rate
- Changes in coordination and mobility

Simply said, Jarisch-Herxheimer reactions, or die-offs, exacerbate current symptoms and cause new symptoms to develop due to the disruption of biofilms. Biofilms contain coinfections, fungi, toxins, and yeast, in addition to Lyme itself. These combined results cause numerous negative effects.

Here's the thing: the symptoms you're experiencing aren't just from Lyme. Many think Lyme is so harmful and so dangerous that it is causing all their symptoms. Yes, Lyme can cause symptoms, but Lyme requires a specific environment to perpetuate symptoms at all. More importantly, the severity of your symptoms is often not the result of Lyme. Symptoms experienced during treatment are caused by attacking biofilms with coinfections, candida, environmental toxins, Lyme, and numerous other pathogens and toxins. To kill Lyme, you must expose it. To expose it, you must disrupt and open the biofilm. When you open the biofilm, you release everything inside it, not just Lyme.

Yet individuals usually seek treatment at various centers for Lyme and Lyme only; thus, when they bust open the biofilm and feel the negative side effects (JHRxns), they attribute feeling terrible mainly, if not solely, to Lyme. As mentioned above, fungi (mold toxins, etc.) build biofilms, candida builds biofilms, and coinfections build biofilms. I know I'm repeating myself, but it's important you understand this concept, as it's a crucial reason you should never break open biofilms. Everything is hiding in there, not just Lyme. Moreover, attempts at disrupting biofilms are largely ineffective, whether by natural or synthetic means. When Lyme individuals experience a die-off, they think it's from Lyme. They're not wrong, but they aren't totally correct either. All pathogens, including Lyme, are what individuals feel after a biofilm breakup.

In fact, calling the reaction a JHRxn or even a die-off isn't completely accurate; it's an incomplete definition when it comes to biofilm producing species. Killing pathogens like Lyme, babesia, candida, and so on causes a JHRxn; however, merely exposing them doesn't necessarily mean they're being killed. If they're not being killed, they're not releasing toxins in response to being killed; thus, this isn't a Jarisch-Herxheimer reaction. In the same vein, toxins aren't killed either, so they don't cause die-off. My point is that what you're feeling from breaching biofilms is from both killing pathogens and exposing pathogens and additional toxins. The floodgates open when the biofilm is breached. Not only are you inducing the release of toxins by killing pathogens, (the current definition of a Jarisch-Herxheimer reaction—a true die-off in a traditional sense), but you're also feeling the massive flood of additional toxins, additional pathogens, and more. This causes your brain and body to go haywire; this is what causes you to feel so terrible. Regarding biofilm species, this effect should honestly be called something else entirely. But at a minimum, this is a more complete definition of a Jarisch-Herxheimer reaction in terms of any biofilm producing species. This is what you feel. This is what happens when you try and go after Lyme.

Do you understand why you can't be just a Lyme expert?

More importantly, are you beginning to understand why it's scientifically implausible to try to kill Lyme in most cases?

When you attack Lyme, you are attacking biofilms. Everyone who's seeking treatment for Lyme is experiencing some sort of symptoms, and many individuals aren't prepared for what's about to happen during their treatments. If you and your physician aren't prepared to handle the resulting symptoms and the substances released in association with die-off, then you're not prepared to handle any Lyme treatment whatsoever, regardless of whether you agree with my notions.

Remember to ask yourself "Is my physician capable of treating my Lyme disease?"

What I do know is that our patients get better without ever opening biofilms, without ever killing Lyme. By opening biofilms and generating JHRxns, physicians are controlling the rate at which Lyme and these other pathogens are dealt with. These physicians are, in a way, thinking they know the best speed for killing the bugs. Many times, this causes your immune system to become further compromised and contributes to further symptoms as well as autoimmune reactions. It's almost as if the physicians were suggesting that our own immune systems haven't been evolving and keeping us healthy for tens of thousands of years. I'm all for science, growth, and technology, but to think we know how to manipulate our bodies better than our own bodies do is quite arrogant. We may get there, but we surely aren't there yet.

Remember my analogy about a biofilm resembling a city? Crime is inevitable in any city, but do you punish the entire city - more accurately, do you bomb the city - because of a few disruptions? Do you bomb the brain and body because of the inevitable production of biofilms?

Quite honestly, the real questions are these:

Should I be busting open the biofilm at all?

Are we being shielded by design and by adaptation of our own bodies' ability to protect us from opening the floodgates of the biofilm?

Can I get better without experiencing die-off, without ever directly attacking Lyme?

We've been evolving alongside biofilm-producing species for all our existence, and they were here long before us. It's time we start rethinking our approach to Lyme and to any biofilm-producing disease, for that matter.

Simply said, yes, individuals at our clinic get better without ever bombing biofilms, without experiencing the awful symptoms of die-off, and without ever directly killing Lyme.

Yes, I will continue to defend this position. Hopefully, I'm beginning to convince you why this position is true.

Biofilm: Friend or Foe?

Let me summarize what we've uncovered and learned about biofilms thus far:

1) 80 percent of infectious diseases build biofilms.
2) Biofilms have been around for 4.5 billion years.
3) Biofilms are homes for pathogens that promote survival.
4) Pathogenic biofilms are intricate and well designed.
5) Biofilms are extremely resistant, especially to antibiotics.
6) Biofilms house coinfections, yeast, fungi, toxins, and more - plus Lyme.
7) The existence of multiple biofilm species leads to higher resistance.
8) Lyme exists in multiple forms, not just as spirochetes.
9) Antibiotic treatment for biofilm diseases is ineffective and dangerous.
10) Attacking biofilms results in die-off.
11) Attacking biofilms results in a laundry list of new and old symptoms.
12) New symptoms are a result of biofilm disruption - not just Lyme.
13) Attacking biofilms requires enormous expertise.

Biofilms' Driving Force

Please understand biofilm production is ubiquitous, as nearly all bacteria produce biofilms; it's just more efficient and safer for survival. Just like the homes we build for shelter to promote our own survival, a biofilm is a pathogen's home. Moreover, bacteria have been building biofilm homes for 4.5 billion years!

And they are really good at it. So please, let's stop attacking them. My viewpoint is if they aren't significantly disturbing us (which happens less than 10 percent of the time), let's live with them. That's right: you can coexist with Lyme disease and common coinfections more than 90 percent of the time. This mean you don't have to kill Lyme more than 90 percent of the time to feel better. At Lifestyle Healing Institute, we've proven that after successfully rebuilding the immune system, balancing electricity in the brain, enhancing blood flow, healing the gut and its lining, optimizing hormone function, reducing environmental toxicity and exposure, identifying food allergies and establishing proper nutrition, and providing exercise regimens, you get better. Yes, you must work at these efforts, as well as the mental-emotional connection and lifestyle education, but you do this without ever disrupting biofilms, killing pathogens, or killing Lyme. We get you better in far less time than any other Lyme treatments available. After we successfully diagnose and heal your health issues, it's inevitable that you'll get well. It's not some hippie mentality; it's the facts. Through research, analysis, and individual feedback and data, I've come to my conclusion as stated above. Many people think I'm saying, "Don't disrupt the biofilm; don't kill the Lyme" because I don't know enough about Lyme to simply kill it, implying I just pulled this thought out of a hat. It's quite the opposite; I know so much about Lyme that I know you shouldn't kill it. More importantly, I use a method that's more efficient, more scientific, and less time consuming, which gets you better without the use of pharmaceuticals.

Simply said, you get better and stay better without attempting to kill Lyme disease.

Are biofilms our friends or our foes?

I don't necessarily have a direct answer to that question. I view them sort of as coworkers, with whom we must coexist - coworkers trying to accomplish the same tasks that we are: promoting life by making money, paying bills, providing food and shelter, and contributing to society within their own skill sets. Most of us go to work without disrupting our coworkers' lives even though they may upset us at times. You can't let your own growth, your own health, to be dictated by a coworker. You can't let Lyme dictate how you live your life. You can live, you can thrive, without ever disrupting biofilm species, without killing Lyme.

As I said, we humans have been evolving alongside biofilm producing species for all our existence, and biofilms were here long before we were. It's time for the medical community to start rethinking its approach to Lyme or to any biofilm producing disease, for that matter.

I'm going to spend the rest of this chapter, discussing and proving my viewpoint with sound logic, scientific research, and real individuals' data. Please keep in mind that everything we do at our center is done because it gets people better. I've watched people suffer for months, years, and even decades through never-ending Lyme killing concepts and treatments. Some sold their houses and their properties just to pay for their treatments. They spent multiple years suffering, sometimes out of work. It's just not right, on a multitude of levels. The medical community is failing chronic disease individuals, especially those suffering from Lyme disease. My methodology provides a better way that's proven by the latest scientific research using a multifactorial approach. I'm the first to say that I have a lot to learn, but what I do know is we get you better by doing it this way. We get you better without the debilitating effects of trying to kill Lyme. We get you better without the use of antibiotics and in far less time. We get you better not only in the short term but also in the long term.

Simply said, you can coexist with Lyme disease more than 90 percent of the time. You can do more than coexist; you can thrive without ever killing your Lyme disease and disrupting biofilms. You get better without killing Lyme.

The truth is that it's difficult to beat this type of bacteria, and if you do, there's a debilitating cost (Jarisch-Herxheimer reactions and their consequences). We may think we're smarter because we have a large brain-to-body ratio and bacteria are feeble and microscopically small with no brains. We must be better; we must be smarter. Quite honestly, I've shown you vast similarities between us and biofilm producing species. Moreover, if you were judging intelligence based on the ability to survive, these species would be the smartest by far - the smartest ever. So why focus on killing them?

Biofilm is not a foe much of the time; however, too many physicians view biofilms as the enemy and try to eradicate them and all that's inside them. Some physicians even attempt to starve biofilms of their vital nutrients, such as magnesium, to slow their growth. The fact is, as I've said, nothing wants to die; thus, it comes as no surprise that this causes biofilm detachment in many cases. This detachment leads the biofilm to try to seek nutrients elsewhere and potentially leads to further chronic infection (45). On top of that: starve the body of magnesium? Really? Magnesium is crucial in calming the brain (as you will find out in the next section); it is vital for reactions that generate

ATP (which serves as the energy basis for human life); it is crucial in generating vitamin D and vitamin D-binding protein and the utilization of vitamin D; and it is crucial for DNA replication and repair (67–70). Magnesium is responsible for so many things, I can't even begin to tell you how stupid that philosophy is. Starving the biofilm of magnesium or any vital nutrient means you are inherently starving the brain and body of that nutrient, which causes more harm than good.

I can tell you with certainty that Lyme, mycoplasma, and many other infections scavenge many nutrients from your body, not just magnesium. Hey, they must survive, right? Materials that are scavenged include energy molecules (ATP, ADP, glucose, and more); amino acids; vitamins (especially B vitamins); and common minerals like calcium, magnesium, manganese, and zinc. (This holds especially true for mycoplasma, as it lacks the cellular machinery to synthesize much at all.) You see, these infections will scavenge whatever they need to survive. I'm not sure why magnesium is the one mineral that's often selected as the mineral to starve the biofilm of, but regardless, can you starve the body of basically everything? I sure hope not. You should see how it makes much more sense to replenish your body with these scavenged materials. Replenishing and restoring is much more effective. You're not going to feed the infections; trust me, they'll get what they need anyway.

The question of whether biofilms are friends or foes proves difficult to answer, but I do feel quite often they aren't foes. The best answer is what I already said: a biofilm is more of a coworker, something we can and probably should coexist with. I can, however, make a good argument for it being our friend. Think about it. Since it's well known we've evolved alongside biofilm producing species (as they were here long before us), don't you think we've adapted to coexist with them? Because our immune systems are largely incapable of dealing with biofilms on their own, in a way, I feel it could be our bodies' method of adapting to biofilms. In other words, maybe our inability to attack biofilms is our bodies' way of keeping us safe. If you take this vantage point, our bodies are telling us we don't need to go after these species; in fact, we aren't equipped to do so. Maybe our immune systems can't attack biofilms on purpose?

We can coexist with these species, including Lyme. We must understand the driving force behind biofilms - what makes them tick and how they function - and understand they've been around for billions of years. For example, the number one driving force for biofilm sustainability is pH (a measure of acidity). Also, candida species serve as the glue to bind multiple biofilm producing species together (32). To be honest, apart from our own research, which I'll further explain in Section 4, much of this section is just basic facts about biofilms, because many may not be aware of their fundamental aspects. Many lack a basic understanding of biofilms, yet they feel equipped to treat them, to disrupt them, and to kill Lyme. I honestly don't get it. On top of that, many of these same physicians readily use antibiotics for any infection, including antibiotic resistant, biofilm producing pathogens.

Maybe it took the failure of antibiotic treatments to fully illuminate the vast number of species of infectious diseases that build biofilms - species that have been around for billions of years. Maybe we caused persistent, chronic-disease infections through the indiscriminate use of antibiotics. It's probably a combination of the two and more, but it doesn't change the fact that antibiotics further contribute to our current situation in facing infectious biofilm species. Humans, as a species, are conditioned to destroy invaders we've been fighting for most of our existence. We've taken that external conditioning and implemented it in medicine. The truth is that your body is constantly at war internally as well. Cancer cells are constantly forming and being destroyed; invaders are constantly entering and being tagged and eliminated. We tend to focus on going to war against the invaders by attacking them head on with herbs, supplements, pharmaceuticals, and more, even if it means sacrificing some good troops along the way. That same mentality has carried over to Lyme, despite the noted and inevitable collateral damage.

Simply said, some are determined to wipe out pathogens at any cost, but there's another way. We rebuild, restore, and replenish your brain and body without ever disrupting biofilms, without disrupting Lyme. More importantly, you get better without directly killing your Lyme.

Yes, I understand bacteria have historically been at the heart of many of our world's most debilitating health conditions, and antibiotics have helped tremendously in past treatments. But that doesn't change the reality of where we are today in medicine, especially in terms of infectious, chronic diseases that build biofilms. With this viewpoint, along with our mentally and societally biased conditioning to kill all invading pathogens at any cost, we've seemingly lost sight of the second option.

This second option is to build up the good to properly handle the bad. What I mean is that instead of focusing on destroying harmful pathogens at all costs, we focus on building up the immune system, balancing electricity in the brain, optimizing blood flow, identifying food allergies, establishing proper nutrition, and reducing environmental toxicity, thus promoting a better lifestyle. Promote the health of our own brains and bodies, and let them do what they're designed to do, without attacking pathogens head on and, more importantly, without damaging all the benefits your body can offer. This is also done safely and without the use of prescription medications. You may be reading about this point of view for the first time, but I assure you many others proved this to be true long before I came along. I'm merely broadening this viewpoint to Lyme and many other chronic diseases. What's largely agreed upon is most, if not all, infections enter and develop symptoms in individuals with compromised immune systems. It is also agreed that it's possible to coexist with many of these infections.

However, when symptoms do result, our thought is always to kill the infection to resolve the symptoms. This is usually not successful. Furthermore, the symptoms associated with the infection may not be the result of the infection at all. The probability of this statement being true greatly increases for any type of chronic infection. More importantly, it's especially true in chronic infections like Lyme, so healing the associated brain and bodily systems are truly at the root of improving your condition and alleviating your symptoms. Killing Lyme often doesn't alleviate symptoms, yet it gets all the focus.

You must understand you'll inevitably have many pathogens show up in your system; however, you can undoubtedly coexist with biofilms and with Lyme disease. Lyme, as with all pathogens, is merely trying to survive and isn't the root cause of your ailments. You get better and stay better without ever killing your Lyme.

Simply said, Lyme is usually not the root cause of your symptoms. By accurately diagnosing and treating true underlying causalities, you get better without ever killing Lyme, thus saving yourself years of die-off and hardships.

Three

WHY TRADITIONAL AND ALTERNATIVE LYME TREATMENTS TEND TO FAIL

The most fundamental principle of our healing process at Lifestyle Healing Institute is to use as many modalities as possible of all natural treatment protocols to address as many brain and bodily systems as possible without the use of pharmaceuticals. Because we understand each modality, as well as how and when to use each one, treatment time is greatly minimized. Through vast amounts of research, we've discovered new modalities and refined and optimized old techniques, thus systematizing our approach. That said, none of your previous treatment therapies would surprise me anymore. When you're not feeling well, you'll do whatever it takes to get better, which means trying everything. Some therapies listed in this book aren't bad therapies, nor am I rejecting their scientific bases. I'm saying the concept of rebuilding, restoring, and replenishing is the best way to heal, and other methods are usually contrary to this process. In addition, they take far more time and cause far more symptoms - quite unnecessarily, for that matter.

Killing pathogens like Lyme means also killing part of your brain and part of your body. I find the philosophy of killing Lyme not only inefficient and time consuming but also alarmingly damaging and debilitating. Moreover, it leaves you fearing a disease that countless individuals live with without ever experiencing any symptoms whatsoever. It leaves you with an unwarranted label that sticks to you like glue. It leaves you living in fear of relapse, and rightfully so, because none of the true causes of Lyme were ever addressed in your previous treatments. Breaking away from labels given to you by physicians, and even yourself, proves to be the most difficult obstacle when recovering from Lyme. Quite honestly, the physical abnormalities associated with Lyme are alleviated in a few weeks (not an exaggeration), but the label, the fear, and the stigma linger much longer. Individuals who want to get past the disease and want more out of life drop this label quickly and take off from there. Our experience is that a relapse of symptoms manifests because individuals are unable to let go of Lyme, to let go of a disease they've had for years; sometimes their investment in the disease is too great. Killing protocols (some of which are mentioned below) further instill this fear, this label, and it just doesn't make sense. The time it takes to endure a Lyme killing based therapy is often months, sometimes years, while it never addresses many of the true causes of the disease; again, this only adds to the investment in the disease. Along with the obvious detriments and newly developed symptoms, this is one of the major reasons I reject the philosophy that you must break down to build up - to kill Lyme to get better.

Our bodies are our most sophisticated healing tools; to facilitate healing and growth, we must provide them with what they need. Killing protocols harm our bodies, only further contributing to the damaging symptoms that accompany Lyme disease. We use modalities that are the most efficient, the most scientific, but most importantly, the safest available. Killing protocols cause damage - very quickly in many cases - which creates great risk without much benefit or reward. This is another important reason I'm not a proponent of any type of killing protocol, at least in 90 percent of individuals. Unrefined techniques of current physicians leave individuals with an undetermined amount of risk, which leads to unsafe and ineffective treatments. Moreover, because of the damaging results of prior treatments, we see more and more people coming to our clinic addicted to multiple prescription medications. It takes us a little more time to heal many individuals merely because we must correct all the damage and flat-out mistakes from prior treatments.

Some swear by their treatments, and some have horror stories associated with them. My goal is to inform you about some of the most commonly used therapies in the Lyme treatment arena, as well as some additional treatments that aren't necessarily for Lyme but that many of you have inevitably tried.

There are two major underlying themes behind the failure of many traditional and alternative therapies: they address only one symptom (or one cause, if it's an OK therapy), and the treatment causes die-off, making your symptoms much worse. Die-off requires long, drawn out therapies that make you worse in hopes you'll recover and feel better. I believe in rebuilding and restoring the brain and body, which happens in a significantly shorter amount of time. This promotes healing. Not only do other treatments cause die-off, but when a healthcare practitioner addresses one symptom, he or she has really backed you into a corner. If the therapy doesn't work, where do you go from there? If you put all your eggs in one basket, all your efforts into killing Lyme, then what do you do if you're unsuccessful? Lyme is a multifactorial disease that affects multiple brain and bodily systems, period. The best way to heal Lyme in the short and long term is to address the range of multiple bodily systems in which Lyme symptoms occur.

In this next section, I'll discuss some of the most common therapies that people endure before arriving at our clinic. I'll explain the concept of each therapy as well as the positives and negatives of each treatment protocol, keeping in mind that the overarching themes (and the overarching negatives) among these therapies are their lack of a multimodality approach and their propensity to cause die-off, worsening symptoms. Both leave you further invested in a Lyme diagnosis. In turn, their overarching negatives are our center's overarching positives, because we address Lyme from a multimodality perspective without ever causing horrible die-off symptoms. Let's begin with my favorite: antibiotic therapy.

Antibiotic Therapy

If you've been successfully processing and integrating the first two sections of this book, you know by now that I truly love the use of antibiotics for Lyme, a biofilm producing disease - emoji, emoji. No, but seriously, if you still aren't convinced they're useless in the use of biofilm-producing infections like Lyme (and damaging, as I'll subsequently discuss), your mind is just not open to another way. Or maybe antibiotic therapy helped you personally, and you can't come to grips with the fact that it's not scientifically sound to use it in this regard. As I said, I want people to get better and stop suffering, especially when I know there's a better way. If you got better from any method, whether from antibiotics or from running around a tree ten times a day, the fact that you got better is all that matters. This book provides reasoning and science and, more importantly, a way out for everyone else who's still suffering from Lyme.

What Is It, and Why Is It Used?

The term antibiotics is thrown around and used continuously when it comes to infections, but what are antibiotics, and how do they work?

Antibiotics are a class of medications that act by inhibiting and/or interfering with the inner workings of the bacteria causing the infection. Different types and classes of antibiotics have different ways of affecting the body. They can inhibit enzymes of bacteria as well as interfering with cell wall synthesis, cell membrane permeability, DNA synthesis, and protein synthesis of the bacteria themselves (71).

Whoa, that's a little too in-depth for me. Just tell me how they're useful in treating bacterial infections.

In normal human terms, they attempt to stop bacteria from reproducing and continuing to infect the body. There are many classes of antibiotics that operate with multiple mechanisms for different pathogens, but in the end, they're all designed to disrupt the infection so your body can heal.

However, they also stop some of your beneficial bacteria from reproducing and helping your body (72). It's just the pros and cons of reality. Most of the time, antibiotic regimens are on the order of weeks and months and are uneventful. Quite honestly, antibiotics were of great benefit when they were first introduced and are still effective in numerous situations.

But not for Lyme.

The problem is antibiotics are effective only at treating free-floating bacteria. As free-floating bacteria are usually present in the acute (short-term) exposure phase of many infections, antibiotics can eradicate acute infections successfully. However, in many chronic infections and diseases such as Lyme, the bacteria build biofilms in which they're nearly completely shielded from antibiotics and become quite resistant. (See the entire biofilm section for more details and documented research.)

THE PROS

As mentioned in the beginning chapter of Section 1, I'm writing this book for the 90 percent of individuals suffering from chronic Lyme whose Lyme has already built a biofilm and is shielded from antibiotics. However, for the 10 percent, the acute-phase Lyme individuals (usually the bull's-eye Lyme individuals), in whom Lyme is still mainly in its free-floating phase, antibiotics can be successful at eradicating Lyme.

What is acute-phase Lyme? I classify acute-phase Lyme as Lyme that's established and diagnosed within the first two weeks of the initial infection.

Lyme is a stealth infection, and it's difficult to detect on a test when only 10 percent or fewer of individuals experience the bull's-eye rash. If you fall into this category, however, antibiotic therapy for as little as two weeks can disrupt the Lyme enough without need for any additional treatment.

Now, for the other 90 percent of individuals, the other 90 percent for whom this entire book is written, antibiotic therapy has basically no benefits whatsoever. You may say, "Hey, I got better with antibiotics; how did that happen?" There are two possibilities: either they slowed the progression of Lyme just enough to allow all the good you have in your body to heal and get you better, or you had other infections that you were unaware of that were treated somewhat successfully, allowing your body to heal and get better. Either way, trust me: it doesn't happen often, and you're still left with the damage antibiotics cause, regardless. Now you must heal that damage as well to achieve true, long-term healing; you also must deal with the fact that no other causes of your Lyme were addressed. In the end, both rely on this same recurring theme: we must kill the bad while sacrificing some good and hope the body responds and gets better. As I've stated (like many others before me), why not just benefit from the good in the first place? Then you aren't left with the risk of the overwhelming damage that antibiotics, and most other Lyme treatments, will cause to your brain and body.

Some more experienced physicians use biofilm disrupters/dissolvers to expose the Lyme and other coinfections and then use intravenous antibiotics or natural herbs to combat the infection. In theory, this seems plausible - but not if you understand the true nature of biofilms. Remember, you must be an expert in environmental toxicity, yeast (candida), immunity, neurology, blood flow, and more to crack open a biofilm. You'll never expose all the Lyme, and the remaining biofilm will adapt and become more intricate, more resistant. Your symptoms will worsen, and/or new ones will develop. You may be prescribed medications just to handle your Lyme kill, just because you're so intent on killing Lyme. Just look at the risk, look at the time, and look at the science. There's a time and a place for everything, but not for the use of antibiotics for the 90 percent of Lyme individuals in whom the disease is chronic; they're not beneficial and are outright damaging.

I can even make the argument that Lyme should be treated only in the 10 percent of acute-phase Lyme individuals, because if you fall into the other 90 percent of Lyme individuals, it's usually not the cause of your symptoms.

Simply said, for the 90 percent of individuals suffering from chronic Lyme, antibiotic therapy is not beneficial and goes against sound, modern-day science.

THE CONS

Not only are there barely any benefits from antibiotic therapy in the 90 percent of chronic Lyme individuals, its indiscriminate use is quite damaging and dangerous. As mentioned, antibiotics aren't used for weeks, they're used for months, and for individuals coming to our clinic, antibiotics have often been used for years. Many individuals are prescribed cocktail combinations of antibiotics administered intravenously, often through PICC lines or PORTs, on top of the numerous antibiotics taken orally. This long-term use of antibiotics usually, if not always, causes the following and more:

1. Damage to the gut and intestinal lining
2. Inflammation
3. Immune dysfunction
4. Damage to the brain and neurotransmitter systems

You may ask how this is possible.

Some damage is from a similar mechanism that food allergies can trigger. (Section 4 has more details on this phenomenon.) Antibiotics are destroyers, for better or worse, and it all starts with ingestion. The excessive and indiscriminate use of antibiotics in the great majority of Lyme treatments will lead to gut, or gastrointestinal (GI), symptoms. Antibiotics start by disrupting beneficial bacteria production in the gut (72, 74), then continue to compromise the gut lining, which is responsible for many functions, including helping maintain a specific pH, promoting the absorption of food, eliminating pathogens, and helping ensure the digestion of food so that it doesn't migrate elsewhere, where it doesn't belong (76). In other words, your gut lining and GI system help food properly integrate into your body so you can use it and stay healthy (depending on what you're eating, of course). As the gut lining is destroyed with antibiotic overuse, the gut become less acidic (pH goes up), absorption goes down (malabsorption), and foods cross over into the bloodstream (leaky gut syndrome).

Simply said, the excessive and indiscriminate use of antibiotic therapy to treat Lyme leads to gut symptoms, primarily the destruction of beneficial bacteria, malabsorption, and a leaky gut.

We've now covered the initial damage that antibiotics cause, but how do they cause damage to the brain and immune system?

You may be surprised, but studies have documented the effects of antibiotics on the brain, which include neurotoxicity (brain toxicity), polyneuropathies (weakness, numbness, and/or pain), vestibulotoxicity (balance issues), and many more (73). Unfortunately, most studies conducted don't propose mechanisms for long-term antibiotic use. As with many individuals infected with Lyme, these patients are prescribed antibiotics for months and often years; therefore, it's necessary to illuminate what will happen to your brain and body after long-term antibiotic use. I'm going to take you through a few steps and piece some of these studies together, and hopefully, my logic will make sense to you. My conclusions are the result of my research, our testing, and individual feedback.

To properly integrate the food we consume, our bodies require an acidic environment (low pH) to destroy incoming pathogens as well as to properly break down food to promote absorption. With a compromised gut lining, your gut becomes less acidic and less efficient, making it more difficult to adequately destroy pathogens and break down foods, resulting in malabsorption and many other GI symptoms (75, 76). Moreover, when your lining begins to deteriorate, it causes undigested foods to leak into your blood stream, a phenomenon widely known as "leaky gut" (75). This is bad news. Undigested food particles are seen as abnormal by your immune system, which results in immune dysfunction and eventually autoimmunity (75). With an increase of abnormal food particles in the blood from a leaky gut - the most damaging being gluten and dairy (mainly casein) - there are disruptions in detoxification pathways and immune function, as well as increased inflammation. These effects make their way to the brain, where they disturb brain regions and increase oxidative stress (damage), among other things (77, 78). This leads to inflammation, blood-flow issues, and numerous other complications. Antibiotics cause disruptions in beneficial bacteria in the gut as well as damage to the gut lining/function. I believe that when these two components are disrupted, as with antibiotic use (and especially overuse), antibiotics can easily disturb immune function and brain integrity.

You may think this is overblown, but it's the truth. Moreover, if antibiotics had these effects but were successful in eliminating Lyme, maybe things would be different.

But that's not the case.

And if you ask me, these resulting symptoms are not worth it, especially when you suffer through months, even years, of antibiotic treatments.

Simply said, disruption in the gut lining from the overuse of antibiotics, causing decreased beneficial gut bacteria, further causes detrimental immune and inflammatory reactions to occur in the gut, bloodstream, and brain. This often creates new symptoms or causes old symptoms to worsen. Oh, and you'll still have Lyme.

If you didn't have gut or brain symptoms before treatment, you probably do now. If you already had these brain and/or gut symptoms, they're probably worse. Not only were your symptoms inappropriately addressed, but you also left your physician's office feeling worse than when you arrived (months or years ago, in some cases).

Are your symptoms any better? Of course they're not; they're probably worse. Nowhere in your antibiotic regimen was there a plan to address your brain symptoms, your gut symptoms, your hormonal symptoms, your mind-body symptoms, and so on. And please don't tell me the plan to heal these symptoms was to kill Lyme.

How does anyone think a disease that can potentially represent more than fifty symptoms simultaneously can be healed by cocktail combinations of antibiotics? It's straight ignorance.

Intravenous Hydrogen Peroxide and High-Dose Vitamin C
WHAT ARE THEY, AND WHY ARE THEY USED?

I grouped these treatments together because their scientific mechanisms and therapeutic uses in the body are relatively similar. Hydrogen peroxide's chemical formula is H_2O_2; it contains one more atom of oxygen than water, H_2O. It occurs naturally in the body and can also be found at your local drug store, typically stored in a dark-brown bottle, and is used to clean superficial wounds.

I'd say almost everyone has heard of vitamin C, or ascorbic acid, as it's also produced naturally in the body and is found in so many different types of foods and beverages. When it comes to Lyme disease and its coinfections, hydrogen peroxide and vitamin C are typically used as killers. What I mean by killer is basically a compound or treatment that disrupts biofilms and elicits a Jarisch-Herxheimer reaction, a die-off, or a kill. When used intravenously - the most common method for using these substances in the treatment of Lyme - both hydrogen peroxide and vitamin C are meant to be killers. Die-offs are felt as early as the first treatment. Most treatment centers focus on killing Lyme while hoping for minimal collateral damage. This is often not the case.

Simply said, when administered intravenously, both hydrogen peroxide and vitamin C are typically used as killers. What I mean by *killer* is a compound or treatment that disrupts biofilms, thus eliciting a Jarisch-Herxheimer reaction, a die-off, or a kill.

As mentioned, both substances are naturally found in the body. At low to moderate amounts, both compounds are beneficial and crucial to our brains and bodies. However, for Lyme treatments, both are used intravenously. When used in this way, their potencies can reach a degree that elicits the killing of pathogens, including Lyme. Oral ingestion or supplementation or any other method besides IV administration won't raise the blood levels high enough to cause a kill. Taking ten packets of EmergenC may get you energized and possibly give you some diarrhea (among some other things), but it won't result in a high enough concentration in the blood to kill Lyme or any other pathogen. (Although there are claims of liposomal vitamin C eliciting a JHRxn, which isn't out of the question.)

When these two agents are used intravenously, they become killers. In terms of their mechanisms, they belong to a family I categorize as radicals. This is part of their killing potential. You may have heard of radicals or free radicals and other terms, such as oxidative stress, reactive oxygen species (ROS), superoxides, and many more. Hydrogen peroxide belongs to this family, and in high doses, vitamin C does also; they both cause radical formation (79, 80). These radicals are unstable and highly reactive and are innately designed to kill invading pathogens within our bodies as part of our defense system. However, when radicals are overproduced, as in intravenous therapy for Lyme, they cause major damage to our brains and bodies. This damage includes, but isn't limited to, heart damage (myocardial injury), thyroid damage (destroyed DNA strands in thyroid cells), cell damage (DNA damage), and even brain damage (79-83). One study concluded, "**HP [hydrogen peroxide] irreversibly damages mesothelial and neural tissue.** Although HP appears to have tumoricidal effects...it should be used with caution in humans because of risks of collateral injury to surrounding normal brain" (81). My point exactly - it's not worth the risk. And that study was for brain tumors - obviously not Lyme disease by any means. Do you see any similarities between this damage and the symptoms of die-off that I mentioned previously? Maybe heart damage from die-off can be linked to symptoms of increases in blood pressure and arrhythmias. Maybe brain damage from die-off can be linked to symptoms of brain fog and seizures.

We should be cleaning up radical damage, not causing more of it.

Vitamin C → *Hydrogen Peroxide* → Radical Killing. Radical Damage

As seen above, high intravenous doses of vitamin C turn into hydrogen peroxide, which is used therapeutically to destroy pathogens like Lyme. There's a delicate balance between adequate production (which is good) and overproduction of radicals (which is pretty bad). Thus, when hydrogen peroxide is administered at too high a dose and for too long a period of time, it disrupts this balance greatly, causing killing of pathogens and many of the damages discussed above. This is problematic because many physicians don't understand how delicate this balance can be and thus cause terrible side effects from the overproduction of radicals. This leads to the damage I've discussed. As a natural killer, hydrogen peroxide is one of the strongest. This makes its collateral damage, the most severe from the resulting die-off the greatest, which causes worsening of old symptoms and development of new symptoms. Another point is both vitamin C and hydrogen peroxide are natural substances, and many think since they're natural, they're better, but that's not the case. Many times, natural herbs and substances are more powerful than synthetic compounds. In the end, it's all about the mechanisms; it's about what they do once in the brain and body, regardless of whether they're natural. These are the same reasons you shouldn't use herbs that disrupt biofilms, disrupt biofilm communication (QSIs), enzymatically break down biofilms, open biofilm channels to allow more potent killing, cause immune modulation, and many more. I didn't include a chapter on the use of herbs and essential oils in the treatment of Lyme and many other coinfections because they cause the same reactions. They open, disrupt, and/or break down biofilms, which is extremely dangerous whether you're prepared for the floodgates to open or not. Use this chapter as a basis to answer why you shouldn't use herbs or oils either, because it's all the same outcome. They cause die-off. They open up biofilms. They take far more time than necessary. And they cause you to feel worse. Anyway, if you backed me into a corner, I would use vitamin C before ever attempting hydrogen peroxide, as the negative side effects of vitamin C are far less if it is administered properly.

Simply said, at high, intravenous doses, both hydrogen peroxide and vitamin C cause die-off. They can successfully eradicate pathogens using radicals; however, the collateral damage can be debilitating, and some may never fully recover.

The bottom line with any treatment administering a killing agent is your physician is manually controlling the speed at which pathogens are killed. When your body is using its own killing agents, its own defense system, your body is controlling the speed. To think we know better than our bodies is just blasphemous. This is one of the major reasons I believe giving the brain and body the tools they need and allowing them to dictate the healing process is the best way to help our bodies build, replenish, restore, and balance themselves. Let's stop trying to tear them down with extraneous control of killing agents.

THE PROS

From a mechanistic perspective, the process of using either of these two agents has some biochemical scientific backing (as seen above); however, expertise on the dosing, the number of intravenous drips, and the negative effects is lacking. My undergraduate economics teacher once told me that one of the fundamental aspects of economics is "Good intentions do not necessarily mean desirable outcomes." This is the case when it comes to intravenous hydrogen peroxide and/or vitamin C therapy. The thing is both intravenous hydrogen peroxide and vitamin C treatment, at the right dose, can truly be healing and have been used for decades in various modalities.

Hydrogen peroxide is used for post–heart attack therapy. It's been used to increase blood flow by increasing oxygen delivery. Being one of strongest killers, hydrogen peroxide can successfully kill a substantial number of pathogens. It works especially well for pathogens located outside the cell (extracellular), and I would recommend this therapy hands down before antibiotics because at least it has science on its side; at least it does something. But the collateral damage of hydrogen peroxide therapy is so extreme that it makes use of this method virtually obsolete in our center as a tool for our Lyme individuals.

High-dose or megadose intravenous vitamin C therapy has been used for cancer treatment. It was brought to light by Nobel Prize winner Linus Pauling when he proved in a case study that an intravenous infusion of ten grams of vitamin C could extend cancer patients' lives six fold. Some of the latest research shows evidence that high-dose intravenous vitamin C therapy has a positive effect on disease duration and reduction of viral-antibody levels.

Somehow these dosages, durations, and understandings have been lost, which is a pattern I've seen frequently in many therapies. The older research is often great; however, over time, this sound logic and reasoning are lost, making the current therapies ineffective and dangerous. Quite frankly, many physicians don't put in the necessary research to truly understand how to use certain modalities of treatment.

THE CONS

As stated numerous times, hydrogen peroxide and vitamin C are two of the most potent killing agents you can find. This makes their damaging collateral effects some of the worst you'll encounter. So, that I don't repeat myself further, go back a couple of pages and look at the possible damage that can happen as early as the first treatment. When it comes to attacking Lyme using killing agents, it's not whether you'll get die-off symptoms; it's when and how bad will they be. Whether you come down with the flu; you're kneeling over the toilet, puking your guts out; your joints are beginning to ache; or you feel as if your body and brain were on fire as you stare at the wall at four o'clock in the morning, trying to get a few hours of poor-quality sleep, die-off symptoms attack your already fragile brain and immune system. Trust me: it's not whether but when and how bad. I know many can attest to these results. On top of you feeling so terrible, it's now months later, and you've been forced to rebuild your body with rest and hope it responds in a positive manner. I'm sorry that this has happened to you.

Simply said, when attacking Lyme with a killing agent, such as hydrogen peroxide or vitamin C, it's not whether you get die-off symptoms; it's when and how bad they'll be. When it comes to hydrogen peroxide treatment, the die-off symptoms are some of the worst you'll ever experience.

Ozone and Hyperbaric Oxygen Therapy
WHAT ARE THEY, AND WHY ARE THEY USED?

I'm repeating myself because I want you to understand where I'm coming from and how I arrived at my conclusions and viewpoints on these topics. As with most therapies (except for antibiotics for Lyme treatment), each therapy has good scientific backing. However, the common theme is risk versus reward. With protocols that elicit a kill, the risk is just too great, especially when you're left to pick up the pieces for weeks, months, or even years thereafter. This comes after killing for months and months, suffering almost every day during the "healing" process.

Ozone and hyperbaric oxygen therapy (hyper means elevated; baric means pressure) are two more of these treatment options many people with Lyme will try. Both ozone and hyperbaric oxygen therapy increase oxygen uptake and use in the body. Poor blood flow is a symptom of almost every chronic disorder, including Lyme disease. To simplify things, blood flow is the ability of your blood and lymph (circulatory) system to deliver nutrients and remove waste. As your Lyme and accompanying symptoms begin to degrade your body, blood flow inevitably becomes compromised. One way to increase blood flow is to increase oxygen use throughout the body. This is basically the thought process behind ozone and hyperbaric oxygen therapy.

Each process is a bit different, but ozone therapy usually begins by sweating the individual to open the pores to increase uptake of ozone. The next step is to use a salt to dry the skin and subsequently administer the ozone with dry skin and open pores. It can be administered using various techniques, dosages, and entry points. Hyperbaric oxygen therapy uses an enclosure that increases air pressure. This increased pressure creates a driving force that pushes more oxygen than normal into the body. Typically, a hyperbaric chamber operates at about 1.8 to 2.3 atmospheres; the pressure at sea level is about 1 atmosphere.

Simply said, hyperbaric oxygen and ozone therapies have good scientific backing; however, improper use results in killing through radical generation with treatment often being too long and inefficient.

THE PROS

Both therapies will increase oxygen in the body, which has been shown to have a multitude of positive correlations. Hyperbaric oxygen therapy (HBOT) involves breathing oxygen in a pressurized chamber. The Food and Drug Administration (FDA) has cleared hyperbaric chambers for certain medical uses, such as treating decompression sickness suffered by divers (122). The treatment also has many other pertinent uses ranging from headaches and exercises recovery to chronic diseases such as Lyme, although these uses are not approved by the FDA. Ozone therapy has been used in Europe for decades, and I know many physicians swear by these treatments because they've seen positive effects for many conditions. Blood flow is a tremendous concern among Lyme individuals and must be corrected to ensure proper healing. These treatments are aimed at correcting this deficiency as well as other abnormalities. Quite honestly, if they were done properly, I'd be a strong advocate of these therapies, but often they make individuals feel worse. Much of the proper technique is seemingly lost, which only hurts the individuals receiving treatment. It's a shame because science has shown how beneficial they could be if done properly. If you backed me into that same corner again, I'd choose hyperbaric over ozone therapy for the same reasons stated earlier. Vitamin C is safer than hydrogen peroxide, and hyperbaric is safer than ozone—that is, if done properly.

THE CONS

The cons, as with the majority of these alternative treatments, stem from the fact that they easily cause die-off symptoms. I don't believe people need to experience die-off to heal, to feel worse in hopes of feeling better. Increased oxygen is a great tool for healing blood-flow issues; however, if oxygen levels get too high, radicals will be generated, thus promoting die-off and damage to the brain and body. I've seen it, heard about it, and researched it. I could discuss additional therapies aimed at increasing blood flow and detoxifying the blood, such as ultraviolet blood irradiation, but that would just be redundant.

The bottom line is that these treatments require several weeks or even months, further increasing the probability of die-off symptoms. The risk is just too great. Moreover, they address only one aspect of Lyme symptoms; these therapies frequently fail to use a multifaceted approach.

This doesn't mean our center won't address your blood-flow issues. Not only do we understand the complex mechanisms involved in diagnosing and correcting blood flow, but we also do so without causing die-off symptoms. More importantly, blood flow is just one issue that's contributing to your symptoms. If either or both therapies are successful, that still doesn't ensure healing, especially in the long term, as there are a bevy of other causes and symptoms contributing to your Lyme. One tool can't lay the foundation to restore your body back to normal health. Lyme requires a multifactorial, multitool approach that gives your brain and body the best chance to heal.

Simply said, oxygen therapies have good scientific backing and great therapeutic advantages; however, they're similar to high-dose vitamin C and hydrogen peroxide therapy because the risk of eliciting a kill is too great, often because their proper uses have been distorted over the years. A kill causes symptoms to worsen, which doesn't help you rebuild, restore, and heal your Lyme.

When it comes to Lyme disease treatment, individuals try anything and everything to feel better. This desperation to feel better and find answers leads to a medley of different therapies, some of which are mentioned above. Below, I briefly discuss heavy metals, which isn't a therapy aimed at killing Lyme, but I would venture to guess you've tried this therapy. Many attribute their symptoms to heavy metals, so I wanted to address this topic to help you understand why this treatment didn't probably did not alleviate your symptoms.

Heavy Metals

Treatment for heavy metals is one of the most common alternative therapies discussed and used in centers across the United States. To affect your health, heavy metals must be present at tremendously high levels. Continuous exposure to a high level of metals over a prolonged time frame quickly causes detrimental health ailments. For most individuals suffering from chronic Lyme disease, heavy metals aren't the underlying cause and usually aren't a large contributing factor.

Some individuals emphasize the possibility of heavy metal exposure because their prior physicians, their biological dentists, and their own research emphasized possible infections and/or mercury or heavy metal exposure. Since heavy metals are usually not overlooked, especially when it comes to numerous years of failed treatments of Lyme individuals, heavy metals are usually addressed prior to an individual's arrival at our center. More importantly, individuals coming to our clinic for treatment don't feel better with most, if not all, of their heavy metals removed. Please understand that heavy metals are like toxins from the environment in that removing the source is usually not enough to initiate healing. You must remove the source and correct the damage to the brain and body that has inherently ensued. This is the most crucial and overlooked step when addressing heavy metals as well as other types of toxicity. Additionally, your exposure to environmental toxins is usually greater and much more damaging than your exposure to heavy metals.

If you're suffering from Lyme, either your heavy metals were already addressed, your exposure was minimal, or the resulting damage was never addressed. Regardless, you still don't feel better, which proves the metals aren't the underlying cause of your illness. So, next time you're told to remove those mercury fillings and everything will be OK, please be skeptical. (But I'd still remove them anyway.)

Simply said, heavy metal toxicity is usually not the underlying cause of your Lyme and usually isn't even a large contributory factor. Our emphasis is on environmental/industrial toxicity as having the highest probability for the most damaging toxicity effects on the brain and body.

Four

A Multifactorial Approach: What We Do Differently

We see individuals every day who are struggling to keep their heads above water. They tend to make great dietary choices and have high health IQs, yet it's been several years since they've felt like themselves. Any little change, whether it's a food choice or light exercise, causes an immediate debilitating response, which leaves them spending the next few days recovering from previous and/or new symptoms. After numerous treatments at numerous health centers, no one can figure out what's going on. At Lifestyle Healing Institute, we specialize in patients like you - people whose prior physicians have said, "I'm not sure why this isn't working; this therapy works for 95 percent of my patients." We specialize in the 5 percent for whom nearly every treatment, no matter what's done, seemingly fails.

I'm hoping you've begun to realize Lyme is rarely the cause of your symptoms, especially when you've been sick year after year after year. I've seen Lyme cause preexisting symptoms to worsen; however, that doesn't change the fact that the symptoms existed prior to the Lyme diagnosis. Moreover, the longer you suffer, the higher the probability that Lyme has little or nothing to do with your symptoms. Because this disease spans multiple brain and bodily

81

systems, a multisystem, multitool approach must be used. It seems ignorant to think attacking Lyme will suddenly cause your insomnia to go away or your chronic pain or fatigue to disappear, yet this is what physicians tell you. These symptoms must be managed in a holistic manner, and that's exactly what we do at Lifestyle Healing Institute. We use a multitude of healing tools, which gives you the best chance to heal.

I've spent a lot time researching, reading, and racking my brain to determine a singular cause for all disease. The benefit of my everlasting pursuit of a singular cause is that I've become well versed in the latest research on many different possibilities of disease. Month after month, year after year, I felt as if I were getting closer to the answer, only to be shown it's not just one thing. In fact, it's never just one thing. Disease cannot be definitively tied to one cause for every person every time - at least not yet. Disease is related to inflammation, blood flow, brain imbalances, the mind-body connection, toxicity, and much more. We use a multitool approach, allowing us to avoid plateaus typically seen in chronic-disease treatment, because we continually add more and more pieces to your health puzzle until you feel better. But it's not about just understanding each piece, because each piece of each disease is a different segment of the healing puzzle for each unique individual. It's crucial not only to address each cause and each symptom but also to know how much of a role each one plays in the healing process.

But it involves even more than that, because the order in which you address causes and symptoms varies from individual to individual. Although the tools are crucial to the healing process, the order in which issues are addressed proves to be most important. Many have heard of some, or even most, of our tools, but to obtain optimal results, the order matters greatly. If something is addressed out of order, not only do you not get better, but you could also feel worse. I've designed a protocol that does no harm with an order of treatment that minimizes time and maximizes efficiency and results. Each designed tool has tremendous upside with very little downside. For a clinic - for society, for that matter - causing no harm to individuals during treatment is gravely important. This is the reason the order of treatments is most important.

Every page I've written to this point discusses the science and my reasoning behind why you shouldn't kill Lyme disease, but I haven't told you what symptoms we look for and how we combat the debilitating symptoms associated with Lyme. In the following chapters, I'll discuss numerous tools we use in combating Lyme and many other chronic diseases. My everlasting pursuit of information that helps others has forced me to truly understand the tools discussed below. I'm not detailing them merely because I've read about them once or twice on some random website. I've spent my time immersing myself in understanding each tool so I could understand its usage, applicability, and healing potential. Truly, I can't rank them based on importance, because each tool has a different value to each individual. We're successful because we understand the complexity of each tool, and we know which tools are needed and to what extent; this is something that varies from person to person. Many have heard of some or most of the tools, but not in this light and not as an entire unit with all tools functioning together. Healing isn't just a puzzle; it's knowing each piece of the puzzle (each tool) and the best order in which to put that puzzle together. For example, everyone knows that the gut plays a crucial role in healing, and some clinics spend their efforts trying to heal the gut, yet the question isn't whether you should heal the gut. It's when you should heal the gut, how much you should heal the gut, and so on. And that answer varies from person to person. Not every tool is used for every person; however, everything listed below has been indicated and implemented into an individual's protocol at one point or another.

After I discuss the tools we use, I'll explain in detail real case studies and show how everything comes together. I could talk about the science and reasoning for days on end, but all that matters is getting people better. I'll show you I'm not just blowing smoke; I'll show you real individuals with real results. I could choose our superstar individuals, but that's not reality. I decided to show you different genders, different backgrounds, different cultures, different ages, and different results; that's reality, and that's what I'm going to show you. I could also go into tremendous detail about supplements, brain regimens, intravenous drip contents, and so on, but that's merely a baking recipe; it's merely a formula unless you understand the concept. As stated, these tools change from person to person; therefore, you must learn the fundamental concepts. I want you to understand them.

The Beginning Is a Numbers Game

We run tests for every individual who comes to our center. And we do a lot of testing. In fact, we test more than one hundred different biochemicals to ascertain a true holistic picture of the brain and body. Many physicians and clinics claim to use a holistic approach; however, without testing multiple brain and bodily systems, it's just not the case. By using abundant and sophisticated testing, we truly gain an understanding of how each system is functioning both individually and with other systems as an entire unit.

The tests we run examine the overall function of each system. For example, rather than testing for each individual infection, we test for overall immune function; this shows how your immune system is handling infections and reveals blood flow, GI health, and the brain's impact on overall immune function. In the same vein, if your immune function improves and remains at an optimal level (verified by follow-up testing), we know we've restarted your immune function, and you're now fully capable of fighting most, if not all, infections, including Lyme. This is our approach with all brain and bodily systems. We view them as a whole to understand the relationship among systems and each one's influence on the entire unit, your entire body.

To be honest, we could run significantly more tests, but I founded my clinic to provide true patient-centered care. I know what it's like to be pinpricked time and time again, awaiting doctors for unanswered questions; I know what it's like to be sick. Everything we do has you in mind. That said, we gather enough information to understand what's happening with each individual. I know too many doctors who seemingly guess at what they think is happening. I want to know, as best I can, what *is* happening with your health issues. In the end, I'm an engineer, and I know it's easier to solve problems and provide answers with real, objective data, real test results.

Simply said, we use more than one hundred biomarkers to create a true holistic picture of your brain and body. This allows us to truly understand what's going on with your health issues—no more guessing.

We then pair our testing with past experience, your symptoms, and a specifically designed questionnaire. We analyze the results of this information piece by piece with you when you arrive and throughout your care while at our clinic. This not only allows us to understand what's truly happening, but it also gives you the opportunity to understand what's happening as well. Your educational participation helps ensure your long-term healing.

We have simplified our testing because I'm good with pattern recognition, so I know which brain profiles, amino acid profiles, and toxicity markers represent each disease, each cause, and each symptom. I know what the brain and body look like under stress, under autoimmunity, and under mental-emotional disturbances. After analyzing the information, both objective and subjective, we develop a unique plan that meets your needs to get you better. Many people who come to our center state how they're "unsolvable" and "You haven't seen anyone like me before." I often hear, "Am I the sickest person you've ever treated?" When I hear that, my first thought is how many physicians must've failed you for you to even feel the need to ask that question. We specialize in people like you and finally give you answers to your health problems, thus getting to the cause of your symptoms. Here's a list of things we test for and analyze prior to your arrival. They serve as the basis for our objective data, and we recheck imbalanced values at the end of your care to ensure optimization.

- Neurotransmitters
- Amino acids
- Hormones
- Immune markers
- Blood-flow markers
- Inflammation
- Pathogenic exposure
- Environmental toxicity
- Genetics

Other centers test for additional things, and to be honest, many more things could be analyzed; however, that would be overkill. These are the minimum tests required for a full and in-depth analysis of the brain and body. Sometimes it's easy to get caught up in the numbers, but we never lose sight of the individual; we never lose sight of you. We don't treat numbers; we treat individuals.

I am also aware that many physicians might question the validity of these tests, but I'm not sure why. These same people have not run these tests and seen the results thousands of times; they are usually reading an article someone else wrote and telling you why the test is inaccurate. But that doesn't mean they won't give you their opinions. The reality is just that; their comments are usually opinions. I use these tests in a much more factual and objective manner. What I can tell you is that sick people have sick test results and healthy people have healthy lab values; that is not by accident.

Anyway, you may have a limited understanding of some of these issues, which is the reason it's important for us to explain everything so you understand how you got in this position, what we'll do to get you better, and how this education keeps you better.

Education and Patient-Centered Care

As mentioned above, we discuss your lab results, your questionnaires, your symptoms, absolutely everything with you to help you understand our concepts as well as gain an understanding of how your brain and body function. We'll show you why your symptoms make sense, and we'll show reasonable explanations for them. We'll show you how your symptoms are interconnected, and we'll provide you with the long-sought-after answers that have eluded you. Most importantly, we'll develop a plan that meets your unique needs; it's never just some generic factory formula.

We'll see you every day while you're receiving treatment. I've been sick and understand the process of getting well, the clinic setting, and how I was treated when I was sick. I'll do everything to ensure you don't feel like a number on the wall, your concerns are being heard, and your questions are answered; then you'll understand what we're doing and how and why you'll get well and stay well. For the most part, your treatment program is all inclusive except for a few expenses such as travel, room and board, post program testing, and additional counseling sessions. All initial testing, all initial supplements, your functional neurology program, your exercise/myofascial release program, your hydrotherapy program, your blood-flow regimen, all intravenous drips, and all doctor visits are included.

Simply said, as stated above, we'll discuss your lab results, your questionnaires, your symptoms, absolutely everything with you. We'll spend time with you, listen to you, hear you, and educate you every single day while you receive care at our center.

Without our talking with you every day, making any necessary adjustments to your program would be difficult, and your treatment could take much longer. We move fast and efficiently and make all adjustments accordingly. We limit the number of individuals we accept in our clinic so we can provide the best possible care for each person. Prior to your arrival, we provide you with a free consultation, and we also have an open-phone policy. This means you are welcome to call anytime, as much as you'd like, until you feel comfortable with your decision to come to our center to begin your healing process. I never want you to feel as if we're selling you something or pressuring you to come for treatment. Even after your program is complete, we offer an additional aftercare program that enables you to stay under our care so adjustments can be made, if needed, when you go back home.

The point of this book is not only to provide the latest scientific research regarding Lyme and biofilms but also to show a better way to restore your health. That's why I'm discussing the reasoning and science for the multi-system, multitool, holistic approach that's supported by the concepts in the subsequent chapters. You'll realize nothing is separate, and everything is interconnected.

Simply said, I founded this center to provide true patient-centered care. Everything is done with you in mind; I want you to feel safe, and I want your input before, during, and after your care.

The Mental-Emotional, Mind-Body Connection Emotional Intelligence

With all the science and numerous physical and physiological tools needed to combat Lyme, it's sometimes easy to forget one of the most basic and crucial tools of healing, which is the mental-emotional, mind-body connection. I don't mean to offend anyone, however, some may find this section somewhat insensitive or harsh, but I assure you it's the truth. Please read this section with an open mind, and take a step back and ask yourself whether any of these statements apply to you. This section isn't meant to downplay your symptoms by any means. This isn't meant to imply your issues are mental and you don't have real physical symptoms. Most of this book is spent discussing the science and the physical abnormalities behind Lyme, so I know they're real issues. I want you to understand that any chronic disease, especially Lyme, also has deep-rooted issues that lie elsewhere. We'll help you with these issues, and after you address them appropriately, there's no looking back; nothing can stop you.

You must be your own biggest healer and take some responsibility for your disease, and most of all, you must truly want to get better. That may sound harsh, but ask yourself that very question: Are you truly ready to get better? This is the first and most important step to healing any disease. You must commit to taking hold of your own health and becoming your own biggest advocate. The longer you're sick, the more time you invest, the more your family members invest, the more money you invest, and the more you invest in being sick.

I've watched individuals transform physically yet remain stagnant mentally. Their lab results improve, their objective examinations improve, and even their own lists of symptoms shrink, but their perceptions of their diseases remain. They get hyperfocused on the symptoms that remain and lose sight of the progress they've made; they lose sight of symptoms that have diminished. Sometimes close family members fall into this cycle and contribute to their mental stagnation. It's truly heartbreaking to observe, because they're so close to getting better; however, some individuals are just not ready or able to get better. We get you better, and I'm telling you this only because it helps you through this process, and it wouldn't do you justice if I didn't mention the mind-body component in healing. All healing is done by you. We are facilitating your healing by understanding the complexity of your disease and which tools you need to get better; however, in the end, your body does all the work. During and after our treatment, if you can't see your body getting healthy, your labs improving, and your symptoms diminishing, then you truly must look at yourself as part of the problem. You may have very real issues that aren't caused by something external, something physical, but are caused by you - by your mind.

You must ask yourself if you ready to let go of your investment in being sick.

Are you truly ready to get better?

The mind is so powerful it can keep you stagnant despite vast amounts of improvement. You may think these statements sound nothing like you, but if you have a label of a chronic symptom or chronic disease like Lyme, you are inherently attached to the label. Anyone who has a chronic disease or chronic symptom like chronic fatigue, chronic pain, or chronic migraines also suffers from chronic mentality syndrome. In other words, if your mind is unhealthy, your perception of yourself is unhealthy. If you believe you have pain, you have pain; if you believe you are sick, you are sick. As we correct your medley of physical/physiological abnormalities, your mind must be ready to drop the labels and accept the improvement. If you continue to believe symptoms are there when your objective labs have improved, you need to look at yourself as a possible part of your disease; you need help obtaining a healthy mind. If you continue to believe symptoms are there when your objective labs have improved, and you quickly jump to a new physical and external possibility, you need help obtaining a healthy mind.

An individual in our care was "disappointed nothing was abnormal with test results" after the results came back from an extensive follow-up lab panel. The individual was looking for something concrete that explained their remaining symptoms. The mind is unbelievably powerful and can cause very real pain, very real fatigue, and very real symptoms, yet the disease, the physical abnormality, may no longer be present. As I've said, this doesn't mean you don't have real, objective symptoms and abnormalities upon arrival, but we heal those issues. I'm referring to when your lab work begins to improve, the color in your face returns, you're now exercising, and you're now sleeping, but you still believe you have a laundry list of symptoms - you still believe you're sick. Often, simple improvements are all you need to return to your life; sometimes that doesn't happen, but it occurs approximately 20 percent of the time for individuals at our clinic. For the great majority, we reteach your brain, your body, and your mind to be healthy. We heal your brain and body as we help you obtain a healthy mind and a healthy perception of the world and of yourself. By obtaining the tools needed for a healthy mind, anyone can achieve long-term healing.

It may sound ridiculous, especially when you're suffering from a debilitating disease, but this proves to be an extremely difficult step, and many get defensive when we try to broach many of these topics. Through years of suffering and doctor after doctor attaching more and more labels to you, you even attach labels to yourself. Once you identify with a label, a disease, or a symptom, you're losing the battle within your own mind (your mental-emotional, mind-body connection).

To be honest, it's hard to blame you for this. Nearly every doctor has failed you, and you're getting sicker by the day with no end in sight. Sick has become normal to you, and you've forgotten what it's like to feel good. I understand how easy it is to lose faith in the physicians providing your care as well as to lose faith in yourself.

But you can't.

And yes, that's easy for me to say, but you can't.

Simply said, you must take hold of your own health and become your own biggest advocate. You are your biggest healer.

Addressing deep-rooted emotional issues enables you to attain long-term healing. We heal your physical issues in a matter of weeks (and I'm not exaggerating), but without a high level of emotional awareness, you will find it difficult to see the result you're expecting. Our experience is that the relapse of symptoms is directly correlated with how much of the mental and emotional work that you're willing to do. We've concluded that, after leaving our center, individuals who truly take off and achieve great heights in their healing process put in the necessary emotional work essential to their long-term healing. Individuals who don't do the necessary emotional work usually fail to meet their long-term healing goals. We help you with this aspect of your healing process. We provide tools that fit within your own framework, your own belief system. For example, meditation is one of the best tools there is for mindfulness, relaxation, and healing, but it may not fit your belief system, and that's OK. If you let down your guard, we can help you regardless of your belief system. We help you uncover, discover, rediscover, and develop your own core values. With Lyme, there's no one-size-fits-all method, especially when it comes to the mind-body connection.

Simply said, we help you in every way possible, which means helping you physically, physiologically, mentally, and emotionally. Lyme requires a multisystem approach, and this is another tool that's crucial in your healing process.

I've seen firsthand how difficult it is for people to let go of their Lyme disease stigma. When I speak to our Lyme individuals and ask them about their symptoms, many say, "I have the insomnia. I definitely have the brain fog and the joint pain." You don't have *the* joint pain and *the* insomnia from *the* Lyme; you have insomnia and joint pain. Regardless of whether you agree with my view that these symptoms (and nearly all other symptoms) aren't from Lyme, you can't possibly think every symptom is caused by Lyme disease. In some respects, whether consciously or subconsciously, you let Lyme become a part of your identity. This doesn't change the fact that you must let go of Lyme disease to achieve your healing goals, but we also realize you need help with this important part of your healing protocol. That's why our protocol provides you with numerous counseling sessions with our mind-body specialist, who has more than thirty years of experience. Our counselor takes your healing expectations to new heights, heights that aren't reachable by addressing only physical abnormalities. When you drop the label or stigma of Lyme, you finally become capable of moving on from the disease so you'll no longer live in fear of it. If you harness your own core values within your own unique framework, no disease will take hold of you again. Most individuals with Lyme are invested in the disease not only financially but also mentally. The longer you suffer, the more the suffering becomes your norm. We've even had individuals relate Lyme to cancer; that's how strongly they feel about and identify with the disease. We change that mind-set, both physically and mentally.

Mentally, you may not be ready to let go of Lyme, to let go of the symptoms you've suffered for a long time. But you must let go of Lyme to get well, and we help you do it. Some individuals are reluctant to see our counselor and put in the work necessary for long-term healing, but addressing and developing mental and emotional tools is one of the most crucial steps in healing; I cannot state that enough. When you wake up in the morning and you're comfortable in your body, you're happy with yourself, those idealities last a lifetime. If you continually seek help or focus on this symptom or that symptom, your healing will be only temporary. True healing takes place within you.

As I've said, this discussion isn't meant to diminish the real physical and physiological symptoms you're experiencing. Lyme and its symptoms suck. Yet, as I've stated numerous times, Lyme requires a multisystem, multitool approach, and to neglect the mental and emotional component of any disease isn't fair to you.

These few paragraphs just scratch the surface behind the mental-emotional, mind-body realm, but this must be said. In no way does this chapter insinuate that we will judge you, put you in some category, or anything of that nature. I established this center to provide true patient-centered care, to spend time with each one of you. We care tremendously about getting you better, and the mind-body connection is impossible to ignore in any chronic disease, including Lyme. I know what it's like to be sick, and I know what it's like to feel better. You, as an individual, become much stronger after going through all this; you become much stronger when you leave Lyme behind. My hope is these words resonate with you and you will reflect on what I'm saying. Healing is a team effort. We support you physically, physiologically, mentally, and emotionally. Letting go of Lyme and the inherent investment in the disease is one of the hardest things you'll face during the healing process. Once you achieve it, there's no turning back - ever.

Getting You off Drugs

The case studies discussed at the end of this section are real people with real results. These analyses show the treatment time for each individual. Please note any treatment time that exceeded our initial four to six week program was needed to detox individuals from their prescription medications. These prescription medications ranged from drugs that are easily and dangerously abused, such as opiates (oxycodone, hydrocodone, hydromorphone, etc.) and benzodiazepines (lorazepam, clonazepam, etc.) to medications that are less addicting and seemingly less harmful (like antidepressants, blood pressure drugs, over-the-counter medications, etc.). Yet in reality all these medications mask symptoms and need to be taken every day. In other words, individuals become addicted to their prescription drugs often through no fault of their own but through the ignorance of their physicians who do not understand the true nature of their diseases.

Let me be perfectly honest with you: most individuals will not achieve long-term healing without getting off drugs, whether prescribed or not.

I've watched many lifeless Lyme individuals come through the doors of our center, looking like the walking dead, having tried five, ten, twenty, or even forty or more different treatment programs from numerous doctors and spending thousands and thousands of dollars in their attempts to feel better. To this day, it never surprises me that other doctors prescribe medications like oxycodone, benzodiazepines, fibromyalgia medications, and even ALS drugs (and plenty more), none of which ever get you better.

What's even more surprising is that nobody thinks these individuals are addicted to medications, even the individuals themselves. We must get you off your medications, whether prescribed or not, for you to achieve long-term healing.

I don't want to sound as if I am putting down drugs, surgeries, or anything of that nature; these things have saved countless lives, including my own. I believe there's a proper time and place for everything, including the use of prescription drugs when necessary. Moreover, drugs sometimes provide confidence that symptom reduction is possible, and they allow your body to accept our treatment during the initial phases. This is often the reason we leave you on your drugs until we address the true causes of why you needed them and had to go on them in the first place. On top of that, drugs have specific mechanisms in the brain and body. If they are understood, they show where your abnormalities are and what is helping to resolve them, even if what is helping is a drug. This allows us to address these issues naturally as well as addressing the true cause of your addiction to get you off drugs in a short amount of time while minimizing withdrawal symptoms.

Simply said, yes, drugs are needed in some short term situations, but not in our treatment and not for the overwhelming majority of Lyme individuals.

Drugs have many problems. Besides their many detrimental effects, which are discussed below, I find one of the biggest problems with medications is they're designed for the short term. In many cases, your physician isn't equipped to handle your symptoms—thus, the use of medications. Many prescription medications used in other Lyme treatments aren't meant to be taken every day for months, even years on end. Not only were your symptoms mismanaged, but now you're taking drugs every day, and you still don't feel better.

In the large majority of cases, medications are no longer helping anymore, as they provide merely one hour of relief during the day, an hour during which you feel somewhat normal. If you feel normal while on drugs, it means you feel abnormal without them; this isn't your fault, and we'll change that perception. I also understand medications provide a mental and physical safety net, so if all else goes wrong, at least you have your medication to get through the day. Trust me: we help you through this process. You may be perceived as being less of a person and lacking moral character by others, and sometimes even by yourself, because of your medications - medications prescribed by an inadequate physician who doesn't understand the brain at all. Let me be blunt: Lyme physicians, you're not helping. You're making the situation worse.

Quite honestly, it doesn't matter whether you're on drugs to cope with an emotional trauma, or maybe you've made some poor choices, or maybe you have a diagnosed condition from a physician who prescribed you medications. Regardless, it doesn't matter. We help you through this process.

Yes, there's a time and place for everything, and I'm not suggesting everyone's on drugs, nor do I mean to group everyone into one category; however, this topic must be discussed. For the great majority of people, getting off medications is absolutely necessary.

To be a Lyme expert, you'd better be good at drug detoxing. No surprise here, as you also must be an expert on immune issues, GI issues, neurological abnormalities, blood-flow concerns, mental-emotional blockages, and many more issues, because healing is multifactorial. Most agree that symptoms are multifactorial (i.e., stem from multiple issues); therefore, we use a multifactorial approach to get individuals better. My frustration is with our medical society, which doesn't know how to handle this disease or how to handle your symptoms. If it did, the disease wouldn't be much of a problem. I want people to read this book so they understand that kind of thinking is wrong. I realize you often feel uncomfortable when your doctor says he or she is going to put you on a medication. You're right to feel that way, because it merely serves as a short-term solution at best.

Simply said, getting off drugs is a crucial step in ensuring long-term healing. We detox you off your medications with minimal withdrawal symptoms by truly addressing the underlying causes of your addiction while treating you with the utmost respect that you deserve.

Relapse is a part of recovery at traditional rehab centers because they fail to understand drugs and addiction from a neurological and physical perspective; this is just a sad excuse for not truly understanding the science behind addiction. Trust me: relapse isn't part of recovery.

If you go to any Lyme center or any chronic-disease center, they must understand how to get you off drugs safely. I can't emphasize enough how important this step is in achieving long-term healing. If you made it past the first few physicians without masking your symptoms with medications, then you're doing very well. The problem is that many Lyme centers and Lyme experts are using drugs to combat horrible die-off symptoms, leaving their patients addicted to terrible drugs like Lyrica*, Xanax*, Klonopin*, Ativan*, Trazodone*, Rilutek*, antidepressants (SSRIs, etc.), opiates, and more. It's horrible to witness, because it's so easily avoidable. Many individuals come to our clinic addicted to numerous medications through no fault of their own, and it's painful to see, because it's so unnecessary.

Simply said, many Lyme experts put you on drugs to combat inevitable, horrifying die-off symptoms. Even if you get better under their care, you're left addicted to harmful medications you eventually must stop to achieve long-term healing.

We change your situation and get you off medications quickly, safely, and without your suffering through the withdrawal process.

You're not addicted to drugs; you're addicted to the effects of the drugs. We stop those effects safely and all naturally. I'll touch on this in later chapters, but I must explain the brain and why individuals seek relief from medications in the first place. In the brain, regions can be either overactive, underactive, or balanced. If you suffer from an overactive or underactive brain, you tend to find relief from medications. What I mean by an overactive brain is a brain that suffers from too much electricity. Conversely, what I mean by an underactive brain is a brain that suffers from too little electricity. Drugs change electricity in many brain regions, which causes individuals to feel more balanced. Now, this feeling is only temporary; therefore, we address the true cause of the neurological electrical imbalance. The type of drug you find relief from provides us with much needed information to find the imbalance.

Symptoms of an overactive brain are insomnia, chronic pain, anxiety, fibromyalgia, poor blood flow, high blood pressure, heart arrhythmias, motor and coordination issues, and more; these are symptoms Lyme individuals experience every day. Medications such as opiates, benzodiazepines (Xanax˚, Klonopin˚, etc.), Lyrica˚, blood pressure medications (both alpha and beta blockers), and more calm your overactive brain, which is the reason they are prescribed.

Symptoms for an underactive brain are chronic fatigue, depression, brain fog, ADD/ADHD, mobility and coordination issues, poor blood flow, and more—yet again, symptoms Lyme individuals experience every day. Medications such as stimulants (Vyvanse˚, Addcrall˚, cocaine, etc.), some antidepressants (SSRIs - Zoloft', Paxil', Lexapro', Cymbalta', etc. - and MAOIs), and more help stimulate your underactive brain, thus helping to relieve your symptoms.

These are reasons you feel better, at least temporarily, while on drugs, and that's why so many physicians prescribe them. Moreover, most symptoms worsen or initially develop when you attempt to kill Lyme, because killing Lyme disrupts electricity in the brain. The most "experienced" Lyme centers use multiple medications to resolve your worsening symptoms, which are inevitable when undergoing die-off from Lyme treatment.

But those same doctors never get you off the medications they initially prescribed to you. (Not to mention that you shouldn't try and kill Lyme, anyway.)

Many doctors lack a true understanding of Lyme and its symptoms, including drug addiction. And yes, one of the potential symptoms of Lyme disease is drug addiction. That's just reality, and it must be said. Since the symptoms for both an underactive and an overactive brain are so common in individuals suffering from Lyme, it comes as no surprise that many individuals come to our center addicted to these medications prescribed by their previous doctors.

Simply said, I've spent time discussing medications because it's crucial to your healing process. Plus, when I talk to individuals at our center, they tell me they never wanted to take medications in the first place! The problem is detoxing from medications on your own is too difficult, especially when you're still experiencing debilitating symptoms. The bottom line is we get you off your medications quickly and safely.

Most steps (the chapters in this section) are crucial, and you may wonder how everything can be crucial.

Because everything is interconnected and because it's important to have a multitool approach for a multifactorial disease that exhibits so many different symptoms.

You must address every symptom using every tool at your disposal.

Anyway, I hope I didn't ramble on too much about this topic, because we have a lot more to cover.

Many are aware of the damaging effects drugs have on the brain, and some are aware of other debilitating, long-term effects of other medications, such as the effects opiates have on the GI system, SSRIs have on birth defects, and many more. Quite frankly, I don't want spend too much time on this subject, but it's important to know that many drugs are linked to debilitating conditions such as autoimmunity, Alzheimer's, disrupted communication in the brain, joint pain/arthritis, and more. Moreover, these are much more common than you think. Obviously, these aren't all the medical conditions affected using medications, whether prescribed or not.

The overarching theme is that medications are designed for short-term use, yet many physicians' inability to understand your disease and your symptoms often leads to long-term use and long-term addiction. As a society, we blame pharmaceutical companies time and time again, but much of the time, medications are being inaccurately prescribed; this isn't their intended use.

Anyway, here's some documentable research you may not have seen:

- Drugs can cause autoimmunity, known as drug-induced autoimmunity (DIA) (85).
- Benzodiazepines can increase risk of Alzheimer's disease by 32 percent if taken for three to six months and by 84 percent if taken for more than six months (86).
- Drug-induced autoimmunity has been known about for many years, dating back to 1945 (85, 87).
- "Drug-induced thrombocytopenia [the autoimmune condition of attacking your own platelets] is a relatively common clinical disorder" (92).
- Joint pain (arthralgia) and arthritis have been known to be induced by drugs (88).
- Antidepressants (e.g., SSRIs) disturb the communication among brain regions as well as between the brain and downstream organs (the hypothalamic-pituitary-adrenal axis, or HPA) (89, 90).
- Chronic antidepressant use can change gene expression of the pituitary gland (91).

Everything Is Made Up of Cells

As seen above, drugs have multiple effects on the brain and body, even on the genetic level. With medicine striving for more intricate and developed mechanisms, we tend to look more and more to the cellular level. Because it's easy to delve deeply into these fields, some fail to see the big picture of how everything functions together, and no matter how scientific and cellular we become, we must never lose sight of the big picture; we must never lose sight of getting people better. However, these days you can't ignore the cellular level. At Lifestyle Healing Institute, we take both the big (overall picture) and small (cellular level) into account because we pay attention to the latest scientific discoveries, which give you the best chance to get better.

Everything is made up of cells; thus, helping those cells will you get better. Makes sense, right?

But where do you start? How do you help the cells?

Our focus when talking about the cellular level is detoxing the cell.

DETOXING THE CELL (CELLULAR DETOXIFICATION)

If you recall, when I refer to detoxing, I'm talking about the elimination of fatty toxins. When it comes to the cell, I'm talking about eliminating fatty toxins as well as cleaning up and recycling the cell's worn-out parts. Detoxification is important, but you must do more than just clean out free-floating, fatty toxins. Think of this process as spring cleaning for your cells.

Now, it's not enough to just expose and release toxins from the cell. After the toxins invade the bloodstream, it's crucial to break them down and simultaneously transport them properly, while supporting the liver to minimize symptoms associated with toxicity. As with everything discussed in this section, nothing is separate, and everything must be considered as a whole unit.

Simply said, we not only detoxify your cells but we also provide the tools necessary for cells to do so on their own.

The Way Cells Talk with Each Other (Cell-to-Cell Communication)

The section on biofilms talks about how many bacteria and pathogens communicate with one another. Your cells are no different. There are great amounts of signaling, stimuli, and responses happening so quickly and so efficiently among your cells all the time. During the healing process, we optimize and increase the efficiency of communication, and one of the ways we do this is through improving receptivity.

Receptivity is a term I use to describe whether a receptor tends to be open or closed. A receptor is something a cell or signaling material binds to, to deliver its message to and/or generate a response from a specific target. For example, neurotransmitters, which are the chemical messengers of the brain, are one type of these signaling materials that are released and bind to receptors. It makes sense to want these receptors to remain open most of the time; however, many important receptors tend to be closed in people suffering from Lyme disease.

Well, how do you open them? How do you enhance receptivity?

There are a multitude of ways to do so, but I don't want to get too sidetracked. (I like science, if you haven't figured that out yet.) However, to understand this a little better, let me go through one of them. As the brain isn't a solitary system, it's no surprise that many cofactors are involved in the biochemical reactions in the brain. A cofactor is something that's required concurrently to make the reaction go. For example, if you are looking at a reaction in which compound A proceeds (converts) to compound B, this reaction may require one, two, or many more - sometimes as many as six or seven different cofactors to proceed. See the example below:

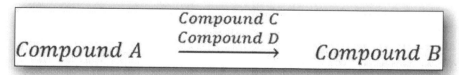

In the above reaction, in which compound A reacts to form compound B, compounds C and D are cofactors of this reaction. Thus, if you are trying to form compound B by increasing compound A, it's vital to increase compounds C and

D as well. Otherwise, the reaction will not proceed effectively. In other words, if you think of compound B as a receptor that requires compound A, compound C, and compound D to remain open, deficiencies in any or all the compounds will tend to cause the receptor to close. This is what I mean by receptivity, and this receptivity is compromised in Lyme individuals. I have found this is the easiest way to describe receptivity.

Simply said, you must look deeper and provide all the tools your cells need. This helps restore cell-to-cell communication and helps your brain and bodily systems get on the same page once again.

THE STRUCTURAL INTEGRITY OF THE CELL

When speaking about structural integrity, many think of chiropractors, adjustments, posture, mechanical links, proper motion, and more, but many are unaware that your cells display their own sense of structural integrity, which occurs both chemically and mechanically. In terms of mechanical integrity, your cells have a surrounding layer known as the phospholipid bilayer, or the cell membrane. Think of the cell membrane as the gatekeeper of the cell, determining what can come in and what can go out. If the cell membrane is functioning properly, nutrients go in and waste is pushed out; this is crucial in keeping your cells healthy. If the cell membrane becomes dysfunctional, cells begin to change shape, allow in harmful toxins and pathogens, and store additional waste. Among individuals suffering from Lyme, this gatekeeper function becomes compromised. Moreover, toxicity greatly affects gatekeeper integrity, making the cells appear ratcheted. You can see this ratcheting below (echinocyte shape) as well as what happens after an individual undergoes die-off from trying to kill Lyme.

Notice how the cells began to change from perfect little discs and clump together after the treatment; this is extremely dangerous and quickly leads to symptoms of high blood pressure, pain, brain fog, and much more. Your ability to carry oxygen and remove waste is greatly compromised, and there's no question that your toxicity levels and inflammation will increase.

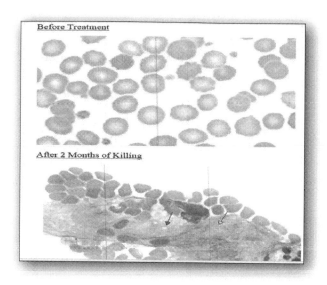

It's important to restore gatekeeper function to ensure the integrity of the cell; however, going after Lyme (and especially its coinfections) leads to even more issues than you had when you started. Not only have you not killed your Lyme, but now you have more inflammation, more damage to the cells, and more symptoms.

Doesn't sound like fun, does it?

Do you see the reason that understanding these mechanisms is crucial to your healing process?

Are you also beginning to see how these issues can be healed without killing Lyme?

Structural and mechanical integrity go well beyond the cell membrane, so let's talk about one more (which is hard for me because, if you remember, I like science). Sometimes, your cells are attached to other cells or surfaces (cell adhesion), which doesn't occur randomly. One of the ways this occurs is through cell-to-cell or cell-to-surface substances, known as cellular adhesion molecules, or CAMs, from which bonds are formed. A genetic condition known as Duchenne muscular dystrophy occurs when a certain CAM, dystrophin, is compromised and the bonds become much more difficult to form. However, these types of bonds can be strengthened, which enhances the structural integrity of your cells. For example, many are aware of the anti-inflammatory effects of resveratrol (COX-1 and COX-2 inhibitor), but did you know resveratrol has also been shown to have uses in cellular mechanical integrity? Resveratrol has been shown to strengthen actin in joints, a vital component in numerous cell processes, including cell movement, shape, and signaling, as well as muscle contraction (93, 94). This is just one example of one natural compound affecting one mechanism in the body. Trust me: there are countless other examples and uses.

It's clear that your cells are extremely intricate, and science is only beginning to scratch the surface of this potential. Stem cells are another great avenue that I won't be talking about, but stem cell research has opened my eyes to the importance of mechanical stimuli. Did you know that stem cells make different end products based on the surface they're placed on (with the same chemical stimuli, I might add)?

Simply said, cells are intricate, but they need healing tools just like every other brain and bodily system. Supporting the structure of the cell helps with many symptoms, such as poor blood flow and inflammation, among others.

The bottom line remains: to ignore the latest cell science is to ignore great potential avenues of healing.

OK, that was a lot of science, but to be honest, it's difficult to write a book that appeals to so many different groups of people. Some of you just want the big picture, but some of you want the science because you want to know why. I truly believe that teaching you what's going on with your brain and body helps you understand your treatment protocol and helps ensure your long-term healing. Moreover, when cell health improves, you can bet the brain is functioning better, the immune system is regulating, toxins are being eliminated, and much more. Conversely, if the cells look as they do in the "after" picture above, you can be sure those functions are greatly compromised. We show what a proper Lyme approach looks like, and we've only scratched the surface of the tools used at Lifestyle Healing Institute. Quite honestly, I've barely even discussed the cell. There are also the topics of cell energy, glucose efficiency, mitochondria, and much, much more, but hey, I'll leave some for subsequent chapters.

The Brain

I'm not going to lie: I like the brain (and science). When speaking about the brain, I tend to use the terms electricity of the brain or brain's electricity. The brain is an electrical organ with about one hundred billion individual nerves (called neurons in the brain) and upward of ten to fifty times more support cells (called glial cells in the brain), which communicate and play off one another like an orchestra. You also have chemical messengers zipping all over the place; these are known as neurotransmitters.

Neurotransmitters are major contributors to the overall electricity of the brain. In a nutshell, you have neurotransmitters that tend to increase electricity in the brain (excitatory neurotransmitters) and neurotransmitters that tend to decrease electricity in the brain (inhibitory, or calming, neurotransmitters), and this electricity differs from brain region to brain region. These excitatory and calming neurotransmitters play a tremendous role in the overall electricity of the brain.

Simply said, the brain has different neurotransmitters that either increase or decrease electricity in the brain. Neurotransmitters are major contributors to the overall electricity of the brain.

We've concluded you must break the brain down by region (by lobe, by cortex, or by hemisphere) and analyze the net electricity in each region because in the end, the brain can either be overactive (too much electricity) or underactive (too little electricity); rarely do we see brain regions that are completely in balance in Lyme individuals. Year after year, the list of diagnoses grows quite rapidly. Yet disorders fall into two categories: overactive and underactive. Below you'll see a list of diagnoses, and hopefully, you see striking similarities between them.

Too much electricity (overactive-associated diagnoses):

- Addiction
- Anxiety
- Bipolar disorder
- Chronic pain

- Fibromyalgia
- Insomnia
- OCD
- Seizures

Too little electricity (underactive-associated diagnoses):

- ADD/ADHD
- Addiction
- Brain trauma
- Chronic fatigue
- Depression
- Obesity

Since you must break the brain down by region, it's possible (and likely) that you fall into both overactive and underactive categories. For example, anxiety often overlaps with insomnia, and chronic pain often overlaps with both anxiety and insomnia - and all of these issues frequently result in fatigue and depression. Sometimes it's easier to see how certain symptoms develop into others; however, it's much more difficult to understand that certain symptoms show the overall electricity of certain brain regions. Your symptoms, in addition to the results from the extensive tests we perform, show us what's going on with your brain as a whole and from brain region to brain region. This enables us to create an individualized healing plan to meet your needs.

Simply said, by breaking down the brain by regions, we're able to pinpoint the cause of your symptoms much more precisely. Our testing, questionnaires, conversations, and experience, as well as your symptoms, allow for this preciseness.

Do you see how it's all interconnected? Do you see it makes sense that anxiety, pain, insomnia, and seizures fall into "too much electricity" and depression and fatigue into "too little electricity"? Doesn't that make more sense than fifteen to twenty seemingly separate diagnoses? I sure think so.

Electricity in the brain plays a major role in restoring overall brain integrity and diminishing symptoms of Lyme individuals. Many individuals arrive at our center with severe imbalances. Their imbalances usually reveal themselves as either too few calming chemicals, such as taurine, serotonin, and GABA, too many excitatory chemicals, such as glutamate, norepinephrine (noradrenaline), and epinephrine (adrenaline), or both. Below is a test result from an individual who upon arrival had too few calming chemicals, serotonin and taurine, and too much norepinephrine. It comes as no surprise that this individual suffered greatly from debilitating anxiety and insomnia. Notice how his serotonin went from 200 to 1,088 ug/gCr and his taurine went from 69 to more than 2,700 ug/gCr while his norepinephrine lowered from 69 to 29 ug/gCr. His anxiety and insomnia subsided in a few short weeks because these values (among others) were individually optimized. Please understand that, because these values are individually optimized, there's not a generic formula for what each value should be. Please don't go and start enhancing these chemicals because you think you know what you're doing and think the supplemental chemicals will get you better. I'm showing this to provide an example.

But what happens when you decide to undergo treatment to kill your Lyme?

After killing Lyme, the brain should get healthier, right?

Your symptoms should diminish, right?

Let me show what happens when you decide it's beneficial to undergo treatment to kill your Lyme. The values underneath the bold-faced values (in gray) are this individual's neurotransmitters just a few weeks prior. For example, you see this individual's glutamate (the most potent excitatory chemical in the brain) increased from 45 to 74.1 umol/gCr. Anything over 40 umol/gCr is damaging to the brain, so yes, there was damage prior to the treatment, and it only worsened upon treatment.

	2.5%	20%	80%	97.5%	Result	Collected	Reference Range	Units
Serotonin					1,112.6 (H)	02/04/2015 (6:00AM)	57 - 306	µg/gCr
					836.9 (H)	01/20/2015 (7:00AM)		
5-HIAA					>43540.0 (H)	02/04/2015 (6:00AM)	800 - 13000	µg/gCr
					>43540.0 (H)	01/20/2015 (7:00AM)		
GABA					12.5	02/04/2015 (6:00AM)	2.4 - 12.7	µg/gCr
					8.2	01/20/2015 (7:00AM)		
Taurine					>2930.0 (H)	02/04/2015 (6:00AM)	52 - 1825	µmol/gCr
					2,098.8 (H)	01/20/2015 (7:00AM)		
Glycine					907.7	02/04/2015 (6:00AM)	182 - 2228	µmol/gCr
					1,043.1	01/20/2015 (7:00AM)		
Glutamate					74.1 (H)	02/04/2015 (6:00AM)	6.9 - 73.8	µmol/gCr
					45.0	01/20/2015 (7:00AM)		
Histamine					33.9	02/04/2015 (6:00AM)	4 - 74	µmol/gCr
					23.4	01/20/2015 (7:00AM)		
PEA					91.6	02/04/2015 (6:00AM)	15 - 157	µg/gCr
					76.9	01/20/2015 (7:00AM)		
Dopamine					153.9	02/04/2015 (6:00AM)	64 - 261	nMol/gCr
					101.1	01/20/2015 (7:00AM)		
DOPAC					5,662.7 (H)	02/04/2015 (6:00AM)	360 - 1800	µg/gCr
					1,381.9	01/20/2015 (7:00AM)		
Norepinephrine					52.9	02/04/2015 (6:00AM)	14 - 76	µg/gCr
					39.6	01/20/2015 (7:00AM)		
Epinephrine					14.5	02/04/2015 (6:00AM)	4.7 - 26.8	µg/gCr
					16.3	01/20/2015 (7:00AM)		

Notice how the exact opposite of my first example occurred in this individual; his excitatory chemicals (glutamate, norepinephrine, and epinephrine) increased. His calming chemicals (serotonin and taurine) increased because they were trying desperately to calm this individual's brain down. The attempts were futile, and this individual developed more fatigue, anxiety, and insomnia.

I don't know about you, but I'd rather be the first example, the individual who came to us who didn't suffer through Lyme treatment.

But wait, maybe that only happens sometimes when you try and kill Lyme. Nope.

Notice how these values are even worse than the first example I showed you. Remember a glutamate reading over 40 umol/gCr is damaging the brain. His is 124 umol/gCr after being over 40 umol/gCr to begin with. No wonder this individual's pain increased while his mobility and coordination decreased.

FUNCTIONAL NEUROLOGY

I could go into much more detail on neurotransmitters, but I'd like to touch on a few more topics about the brain. The next topic I want to cover is functional neurology. All doctors, whether NDs, MDs, DOs, DCs, or others, are taught how to conduct a physical and neurological exam on patients, yet many times they're not taught to observe the subtleties from test to test. If you have a trained eye for what certain movements and nonmovements mean, it serves as a basis for a program designed to optimize brain function. Let me give you an example. Close your eyes and put your arms straight out in front of you, palms facing down, as if you were starting the Macarena. Now, take your left pointer finger and touch it to your nose. You just used four different brain regions to accomplish that task. You may think you accomplished that task easily, but under further examination, you may have paused for a split second before touching your nose, you may have moved your arm too fast or too slowly when moving toward your nose, or you may have touched the side of your nose or a different facial feature altogether. These actions (and more) give us very specific information about your brain. The way you walk, talk, accomplish tasks, perform specific actions, and solve problems gives us specific information about your brain. This specificity and preciseness in administering and interpreting a physical and neurological exam is another crucial tool to help restore your brain to optimal health. Brought to the forefront by chiropractors, functional neurology has immense benefits for balancing and restoring the brain's integrity, especially when it comes to motor skills and coordination, balance, pain, brain fog, processing speed, and developmental and behavioral disorders. Notice any similarities between those symptoms and your own? Yet another piece of the puzzle.

But how does this work? When you were performing the nose-touching exercise, you were exercising your brain. After we administer our exam, we determine which brain regions need more exercising than others, which is reflected in your specific functional neurology program. To exercise a brain region, blood flow is sent to the region, and glucose (a sugar that is fundamental in energy production) is used in the region. You make energy (ATP) in that region just to perform that action. Moreover, you build new connections between neurons in the brain, which is necessary for the longevity of your brain. We have a set number of neurons from birth, and all of us have fewer than we had when we were born; however, we do have more connections. Brain activation through these exercises (and just the flat-out use of your brain) builds new connections, which are essential in a healthy brain. However, if your glucose system is inefficient, your blood flow is compromised, and your mitochondria (ATP energy centers) are deficient, brain exercises are not only ineffective but can also be dangerous.

Another point to note is that numerous Lyme individuals present with motor, coordination, and mobility issues that accompany temporomandibular joint (TMJ) pain. Our process shows great success in improving these conditions, thus allowing many of our individuals to return to a normal life that includes no longer needing assistance to walk as well as driving for the first time in years. We've also shown that TMJ pain stems not from Lyme, or any other infection, but from brain dysfunction. More importantly, after we improve your balance, mobility, and coordination, this usually allows the TMJ pain to subside. Often, the brain region that senses pain isn't specifically responsible for TMJ pain.

These are some of the many reasons functional neurology is an important part of treatment. They also show once again that everything requires expert understanding in multiple aspects of your healing process. It also shows how everything is interconnected and why everything must be addressed safely and efficiently. We enhance your blood flow, your energy system, your mitochondria, your metabolic needs, and more, before, during, and after your unique functional neurology program.

Simply said, after we pinpoint what's truly going on with you and your brain, we develop a unique, functional neurological program to meet your needs. This enhances blood flow and energy and thus helps to heal symptoms such as brain fog, migraines, motor issues, balance and coordination problems, and more—the very symptoms chronic Lyme individuals experience quite often.

A LITTLE ON THE NMDA RECEPTOR

One of our most instrumental specialties and arguably the most critical aspect of our program is our ability to calm down the brain and the body, to calm down your overactive brain regions. We calm specific brain regions, which results in better-quality sleep, less anxiety, fewer tremors, and less pain. We remove environmental toxins, which cause disruptions in the brain's neurotransmitters, thus allowing the immune system's signaling to regulate correctly. We calm and regulate the immune and GI systems, resulting in less GI distress and diminished autoimmune reactions. This allows for proper regulation, proper signaling, enhanced blood flow, better digestion and immune regulation, and much more. In terms of the brain, I've shown you a couple of ways this is accomplished, but I can't end this chapter without talking about the N-methyl-D-aspartate (NMDA) receptor.

Remember those excitatory neurotransmitters and those receptor things? Well, here's a little more for you science peeps out there. Glutamate, the brain's number one excitatory chemical in both quantity and potency, is linked to almost every single neurological and mental condition. Therefore, it comes as no surprise that glutamate is linked to acute CNS diseases, including ischemia, trauma, epilepsy, stroke, hypoxia, head trauma, Huntington's, Parkinson's, Alzheimer's, neuropathic pain, alcoholism, schizophrenia, and mood disorders (95, 96). (Again, this list is not meant to be exhaustive.) When the brain becomes too electrified and too overactive, glutamate elevates and begins to bind and activate the NMDA receptor at a much higher rate. When glutamate binds to the NMDA receptor, it causes calcium to enter the cell (96). In a nutshell, when calcium enters the cell (influx into the cell), it causes increases in electricity. This is a necessary process of life and learning, but when this receptor becomes overstimulated, either short or long term, there's a potential for all the aforementioned symptoms and disorders to occur. There are simple ways to help regulate and calm this overactivation and subsequent increase in electricity. For example, magnesium sits on the receptor like a plug, preventing calcium from entering and thus preventing this increase in electricity (68). This is one of ten to twenty different ways we regulate the NMDA receptor.

Simply said, the NMDA receptor closely regulates the overall electricity of your brain; thus, by focusing on this receptor, we alleviate many symptoms associated with too much electricity: insomnia, chronic pain, anxiety, seizures, and more.

These features, this science, separate us from all other Lyme centers. Because hey, the brain is just another piece—a critical piece, and a piece we spend a lot of time on, but still just another piece.

Blood Flow

I mentioned blood flow (sometimes referred to as circulation) in the previous chapter when we discussed the brain. But what is blood flow? There are numerous definitions and explanations, but in simple terms, blood flow is your body's way of delivering nutrients and removing waste everywhere in the body. Nutrients are substances such as oxygen, glucose, and more, while waste includes substances such as toxins, cell fragments, dead cells, and so forth. I use the term *blood flow*, but in reality, *circulation* is much more accurate because it's about your veins, your arteries, your capillaries, your lymph fluid, and all their related components. All aspects must be optimized to promote better flow. Many people make arguments for this cause or that cause, but what's undeniable is that blood flow has a role in every chronic disease, especially Lyme disease.

Simply said, blood flow is your body's way of delivering nutrients and removing waste everywhere in the body. Blood flow is severely compromised in many individuals with chronic Lyme.

It seems logical that, if you can't deliver nutrients and remove waste from your body, you're going to run into some problems, and the longer your blood flow is compromised, the more stagnation occurs. I'd like to talk about veins and arteries and how they tie into blood flow. Quite literally, your veins and arteries get smaller and smaller (these smaller branches are known as venules and arterioles, respectively) until they come together at capillary beds. The capillary beds are responsible for the delivery of nutrients and the removal of waste. This super small vessel system makes up approximately 70 percent of your overall circulation (known as microcirculation), yet many physicians focus on other, tangible large vessels. We easily open up microcirculation, thus promoting flow; however, once again, that's just another part of the puzzle.

We also provide your vessels with tools to expand, we make sure you're exercising properly, we release your muscles, we detoxify your system, and we support one of your primary detox centers -your liver, to handle all these changes. We promote proper lymphatic flow as well, because your lymph nodes are among your hub-monitoring centers. They check out what's going on and send signals to the immune system, helping sort out what stays and what goes. By helping flow, you also help regulate autoimmune reactions in the brain and body.

Many other things significantly affect blood flow:

- Hormones
- Immune system
- Brain
- Total inflammation
- Environmental-toxin exposure
- GI health

Lyme hides in its biofilm, and so do environmental toxins, yeast toxins, and other pathogens. When you crack open biofilms, the floodgates open, and your brain increases its electricity, your hormones begin to plummet, and your immune system becomes erratic, as mentioned in the last section. It's widely known that blood flow plays a tremendous role in healing chronic disease, especially Lyme. It's hard to understand why anyone would ever disrupt this flow by attempting to eradicate an individual's Lyme. I assure you the effects are inevitable; that's what die-off is all about.

In many aspects, blood flow is directly correlated with inflammation. This is especially true when it comes to the size of your red blood cells. Your red blood cells should be about eight microns wide and are designed to efficiently move through your circulatory system, but inflammation can swell your cells to much larger sizes; this greatly compromises blood flow. A simple measure to determine whether your red blood cells are inflamed is a test known as red blood cell distribution width, or RDW. RDW is basically a measurement of how wide your cells are. Below, you can see the impact on the RDW of an individual who has undergone a Lyme killing therapy.

This individual was already high at 15.1 before undergoing treatment, but as you can see, the RDW jumped up to 25.1 after the individual underwent a Lyme killing therapy. That's an increase of more than 66 percent, and the RDW was already high to begin with, and that's only one marker of blood flow! An RDW of 25.1 is an extremely unsafe level, and it's not surprising that brain fog and high blood pressure ensued. Additionally, when the cells jump to such a large size, they begin to clump together. This results in increases of markers in thrombin-antithrombin complex, fibrinogen, and platelets. This results in "thick" blood, making transport extremely difficult. Symptoms resulting from this aggregation include pain, fatigue, brain fog, inability to catch your breath, and much more. You can see how this individual's platelets began to elevate from 268,000/uL to 330,000/uL. I hope you're beginning to see that disruptive issues are not uncommon when an individual is undergoing a killing therapy that elicits die-off. Here's another example of a platelet elevation causing an individual's blood to become extremely thick, resulting in pain and fatigue.

PLATELET COUNT		396	140-400 Thousand/uL	
Platelets		384 High	x10E3/uL	150 - 379

Notice how they jump from 296,000/uL to 384,000/uL. That's an increase of nearly 30 percent, which means blood flow is compromised by almost 30 percent just by this value alone. These are examples of abnormalities in blood flow that worsened tremendously upon treatment. In the overwhelming majority of cases, you don't have to get worse to feel better.

Simply said, many issues are involved with optimizing blood flow, and there's no doubt that blood flow is compromised in many individuals suffering from Lyme. We open up your small vessels and promote nutrient delivery and waste removal, which is an important step in Lyme therapy. Lyme-killing therapies worsen your blood flow, only further contributing to your symptoms.

Do you realize, once again, why it's imperative you not attempt to eradicate Lyme?

There's another way, a better way.

When it comes to a complex and scientific healing process with a disease like Lyme, basic pieces of information are often overlooked. One piece of information is your vital signs, which include markers such as blood pressure, heart rate, respiratory rate, and temperature. By seeing you and communicating with you every day, we're able to monitor these values very closely. Individuals come to our center with heart rates between 85 and 120 and blood pressure reaching as high as 190/120 mmHg. Conversely, many individuals come in with low blood pressures, erratic heart rates, and low temperatures. Many times, it's necessary to analyze blood pressure in both arms. Did you know your blood pressure tremendously affects your body's ability to deliver nutrients and remove waste? Moreover, the blood pressure values in your brain are very different from the blood pressure values taken from your arm; they're lower. Sometimes, this explains why a person whose vital signs show low blood pressure and low temperature has certain neurological symptoms such as dizziness, brain fog, balance and coordination issues, and more.

In addition, many Lyme individuals experience cold feet and toes, cold hands, and a cold nose owing to poor circulation. Others may have purple or pale white finger or toenail beds. Many jump to the conclusion that this a symptom of a low thyroid, since the thyroid helps regulate basal temperature; however, we find it more of a symptom of poor circulation or poor blood flow. Some individuals have toe fungus that doesn't seem to go away even after they apply antifungal cream time and time again because reoccurring toe fungus is often from poor circulation.

There's also another condition known as Raynaud's disease in which, when faced with cold, adverse conditions, your fingers and toes respond by clamping and redirecting blood flow toward the center of your body to your organs. Part of your nervous system sends signals causing this effect. Known as the sympathetic nervous system, it's responsible for the fight-or-flight response, which increases heart rate and blood pressure, decreases blood flow to the GI system, and much more. Another part of your nervous system, the parasympathetic nervous system, is responsible for the rest-and-digest response, which decreases heart rate and blood pressure while increasing blood flow to the GI system. We've found that some individuals don't have Raynaud's disease but actually have poor circulation and an excess of sympathetic nervous system activity. Raynaud's disease usually manifests as many other symptoms associated with poor circulation, such as headaches, GI issues, and more. Please realize how often overlooked, basic pieces of information give you crucial clues to treatment protocols, especially when it comes to blood flow. Sometimes, with an extremely complex disease like Lyme, it's easy to forget the basics.

Simply said, many symptoms are often misdiagnosed, and with a complex disease like Lyme, some of the most basic pieces of information are often overlooked. Yet those basic pieces provide valuable data, especially when it comes to blood flow.

These are important steps in enhancing your blood flow as well as promoting a better healing environment for your body. Moreover, you have a bunch of backlogged waste that hasn't been processed in a long time, and optimizing flow helps the body rid itself of unprocessed waste as well. This step can't be overlooked.

Immunity and Autoimmunity

Autoimmune conditions are on the rise.

But what is autoimmunity?

Autoimmunity is your own immune system, your own brain, and your own body attacking itself. If you are autoimmune, your immune system is attacking you. Autoimmunity includes conditions ranging in severity from allergies and skin issues to more serious conditions, such as multiple sclerosis, rheumatoid arthritis, Crohn's disease, Hashimoto's disease, Graves' disease, and many more. It's estimated as many as fifty million people suffer from such autoimmune conditions; that's about one-fifth of our population (97). Moreover, individuals with multiple autoimmune syndrome (MAS) are classified as having three or more autoimmune conditions, and an estimated 25 percent of people with autoimmune disorders have MAS (98).

Think about that.

Twenty-five percent of people with autoimmune conditions are attacking themselves in three or more different ways. This situation must change. Instead of looking at autoimmunity as a whole, allopathic medicine attempts to slow this progression by attacking the disorders one by one. We've found this process is much slower, less accurate, and less successful than understanding the potential global causes of autoimmunity. It just doesn't make any sense. The fact that you experience multiple autoimmune conditions simultaneously speaks to a global cause, an overarching cause. This also shows that if you're autoimmune somewhere in your body, you're autoimmune everywhere.

Simply said, autoimmunity occurs when your immune system is compromised and your immune system starts to attack your body. Autoimmunity, often speaks to a much larger issue in the brain and body.

There's growing interest and research concentrating on the mechanisms of immunity in general, with TH-1, TH-2, TH-17, regulatory T cells, and other immune pathways being extensively analyzed and mapped out. In a nutshell, there are monitoring cells (such as antigen-presenting cells, or APCs) that roam around and try to tag invading materials. These monitoring cells then grab and communicate to a helper cell (naive T cell) to let it know what's happening. This causes multiple immune signalers (such as cytokines and interleukins) to determine the response your immune system will have (Th-1, Th-2, Th-17, and T-reg pathways). Certain abnormalities generate certain responses. For example, if your monitoring cells find viruses, bacteria, or toxins, this could yield three different responses. If there's a pathogen inside your cells, that yields a different response than a pathogen outside your cells. This is basically an oversimplified version of how your immune system works. If these pathways are continually activated, your immune system goes haywire and starts an onslaught against your system. In a more specific fashion, Th-1 and Th-17 have been shown to play a large part in autoimmunity. Through the latest scientific research as well as our own data from individuals who received care at our center, we have found that Th-17 plays a larger role than Th-1 (in case you were wondering, for all the science nerds, like me).

Let's break this down and simplify it even more. How does your own protective defense system, your own immune system, start attacking itself? How do you become autoimmune?

Through our extensive research, we've found that there are three main contributors to autoimmunity, excluding genetics. (And yes, there are more):

- Environmental/industrial toxins
- Mental-emotional disturbances
- Foods, food allergies, GI dysfunction

They're not in any particular order of importance, as you may be affected by one or all of these contributors, and each plays a different role in each individual. It's not a surprise with Lyme individuals that overall immune function is usually compromised. We've shown that when these conditions are addressed properly, autoimmune reactions are minimized substantially. This causes your overall immune system to improve drastically and function more efficiently.

Simply said, we've found there are three major contributors to autoimmunity (excluding genetics): environmental/industrial toxins, mental-emotional disturbances, and foods and food allergies, in no particular order.

In fact, I've confirmed through our research that there are two major types of autoimmunity: overactive and suppressive. Overactive autoimmunity is your body's initial reaction to one or more of the three disturbances. As your immune helper cells (CD4 cells), your autoimmune ratio (CD4:CD8 ratio), and other immune markers (cytokines, white blood cells, natural killer cells, etc.) begin to elevate, your brain electricity increases, your inflammatory response increases, and much more. Individuals with overactive autoimmunity are usually hypersensitive and react to almost anything different in their lives, whether it's a new food or a new activity, and have sensitivities to multiple different chemicals (MCS). They often get sick with conditions such as the flu, strep, and various other infections.

On the other hand, suppressive autoimmunity is mostly a long-term reaction to disturbances that cause autoimmunity; therefore, prolonged toxicity exposure, extensive food-allergy reactions, and unaddressed long-term mental-emotional issues result in suppressive autoimmunity. With suppressive autoimmunity, your immune suppressive cells (CD8) increase, while your white blood cells, and your CD4:CD8 ratio begin to depress; therefore, you have less immunity and less immune function. In addition, GI symptoms become much more prevalent, malabsorption and leaky gut ensue, the blood thickens, your inflammatory responses slow, and the brain experiences a medley of detrimental effects. Suppressive autoimmunity is worse than overactive autoimmunity. Individuals with suppressive autoimmunity tend not to get sick with infections and usually make the claim "I rarely get sick," yet many times they're sitting in their doctors' offices, so obviously, there is something wrong. They don't get sick with day-to-day infections like the flu or strep, because they literally can't mount an immune response; their immune systems are nearly completely compromised. These individuals usually have more severe issues, yet they tend to report less severity of symptoms than individuals with overactive autoimmunity.

Another note on the CD4:CD8 ratio involves Epstein-Barr virus (EBV). I discussed this virus briefly when explaining the point that only 25 percent of people get mono, showing that most of the time you can coexist with a multitude of infectious pathogens. However, EBV has been linked to low CD8 cells, which tends to make your CD4:CD8 ratio elevated or overactive. Often it's a result of low vitamin D or EBV that's not under control. If symptoms don't improve and this ratio doesn't rectify itself, additional measures should be taken to modulate the ratio to a healthy level.

THE LYMPHATIC SYSTEM AND LYMPHATIC DRAINAGE

You can't talk about autoimmunity and overall immune function without discussing the lymphatic system. The lymphatic system is a network that runs throughout the body and is designed to help the body get rid of waste and toxins. There are hundreds of lymph nodes in various locations in the body, each having its own area of the body to process and monitor. Each lymph node is equipped with its own immune cells to monitor invading forces, cellular waste, toxins, and more. Often, the amount of toxins entering the body and the ability of the body to process toxins are imbalanced, leading to stagnant flow and large amounts of unprocessed waste and toxins. This condition is often seen in chronic disease, especially Lyme. We are always creating waste and being exposed to toxins, and in a normal situation, this load isn't too much to handle. But with excess toxins, excess inflammation, decreased circulation, and the HLA gene (situations not uncommon for Lyme individuals), the lymph nodes become backlogged from being so sick for so many years. If this is the case, symptoms worsen if techniques such as massage and drainage are overdone. Recently, it's been shown that people with genetic susceptibility to autoimmunity have half the amount of lymph nodes as other people. Moreover, people with autoimmune conditions are prone to swollen lymph nodes. This makes sense, because your lymph nodes have immune cells that process waste; the fewer nodes you have, the less toxicity-clearance, monitoring, and processing ability you have. This increases the probability of swollen lymph nodes and thus increases the number of unprocessed toxins and waste, because there are just fewer lymph nodes to work with. Therefore, even healthy individuals can feel sick after a massage, and it's why they tell you to drink a bunch of water after the massage, to help flush out the waste and toxins. Regardless of the number of lymph nodes, a swollen node indicates inflammation and a disruption in toxin and waste clearance. This is also the reason individuals who have cancer often have swollen lymph nodes. On that same note, it's not uncommon to remove cancerous nodes, and many individuals frequently experience swelling and stagnant flow in the areas from which the nodes were removed; there are fewer nodes to process all the waste and toxins.

Many individuals with Lyme disease already make better choices when it comes to diet (no preservatives, food additives, synthetic sweeteners, etc.) and have eliminated most of the obvious triggers (gluten, dairy, soy, etc.). This helps in removing one of the three top contributors to autoimmunity; however, a leaky gut is not by any means the only way foods can trigger autoimmunity. As I've mentioned a few times thus far, macrophages are immune cells that function like little Pac-Man cells, eating invaders if activated and signaled properly. You have macrophages everywhere in your body, including the brain (where they're called microglial cells) and the gut (in the mucosal-associated lymphoid tissue). When you eat anything, good or bad, macrophages monitor the activity and transport the microbes (anything good or bad that can't be seen with the naked eye) via the lymphatic system up to the brain. These microbes have a tremendous impact on the overall function of the brain. If you eat good food, the macrophages transport good microbes, which benefit the brain. Conversely, if you eat bad food and the macrophages are transporting bad microbes, you'll get bad inflammatory reactions in the brain. This causes the lymphatic vessels in the brain to become overloaded, and toxins and waste begin to accumulate in the brain. This is known as neuroinflammation, or inflammation in the brain. Neuroinflammation is linked to numerous conditions, as one could easily predict. Often, individuals with Lyme and many other chronic diseases have enlarged or swollen lymph nodes. If there's neuroinflammation from this mechanism, the lymph nodes around the neck (the cervical nodes) tend to get swollen. Individuals with chronic diseases and immune dysfunction indicate enlarged cervical nodes, which are a direct indication of inflammation and increased toxic load in the brain. Once this neuroinflammation is greatly reduced, neurons begin to build connections and improve the overall function of your brain, like the concept of brain activation and functional neurology. Overall, the importance of the immune system has been gaining recognition in recent years; it has even been mentioned as being the third brain. As I've stated time and time again, it's important to address each system, each organ, and each "brain," but in reality, everything functions together as one unit, one organ, one complex, dynamic system that's completely integrated and interrelated.

If other disturbances are left unchecked, autoimmunity will continue. On top of that, even if disturbances are removed and addressed, your brain and body have taken an enormous onslaught of damage; therefore, it's necessary to heal the damage to restore immune function. Merely removing the disturbances isn't enough to restore immune function. For example, when you clean up your diet, you're still left with overgrown yeast (Candida albicans), a perforated gut lining, and neuroinflammation. The gut must be healed, beneficial bacteria must be replenished, yeast must be killed and removed, and the brain must be drained and its inflammation reduced.

But wait, I have an idea (a bad idea): maybe killing Lyme will fix all this autoimmunity, and it won't cause it to worsen or anything.

Maybe opening the biofilm to attack Lyme won't release more toxins, more pathogens, and more yeast.

Maybe it won't cause more inflammation and more swollen lymph nodes.

Maybe it's not as if you'd attack yourself even more.

And maybe *not*.

Just in case you don't believe that killing Lyme is the wrong approach more than 90 percent of the time, here's an example of what happens when you do so. This individual suffers from an autoimmune condition. You can see how the immune markers (WBC [white blood cells] and CD4:CD8 ratio) increased upon treatment. White blood cells are cells that attack invading cells, while the CD4:CD8 ratio is a measure of autoimmunity. Ideally, this ratio should be about 2.0 ($\pm$0.15) with a CD4 of about 800–1,000 cells/uL and a CD8 of about 400–500 cells/uL. If it's over 2.0, you have overactive autoimmunity, and if it's below 2.0, you have suppressive autoimmunity. See how this individual's values are already elevated and only worsen upon treatment.

Before Treatment   **After Treatment**

TESTS	RESULT	TESTS	RESULT	FLAG
CD4/CD8 Ratio Profile		CD4/CD8 Ratio Profile		
Absolute CD 4 Helper	1473	Absolute CD 4 Helper	1668	High
% CD 4 Pos. Lymph.	52.6	% CD 4 Pos. Lymph.	55.6	
Abs. CD 8 Suppressor	834	Abs. CD 8 Suppressor	855	
% CD 8 Pos. Lymph.	29.8	% CD 8 Pos. Lymph.	28.5	
CD4/CD8 Ratio	1.77	CD4/CD8 Ratio	1.95	
WBC	9.0	WBC	11.3	High
RBC	4.48	RBC	4.28	
Hemoglobin	13.3	Hemoglobin	12.6	
Hematocrit	40.4	Hematocrit	37.7	
MCV	90	MCV	88	
MCH	29.7	MCH	29.4	
MCHC	32.9	MCHC	33.4	
RDW	13.2	RDW	13.0	
Platelets	348	Platelets	447	High
Neutrophils	62	Neutrophils	65	
Lymphs	31	Lymphs	26	
Monocytes	5	Monocytes	7	
Eos	2	Eos	2	
Basos	0	Basos	0	
Neutrophils (Absolute)	5.5	Neutrophils (Absolute)	7.2	High
Lymphs (Absolute)	2.8	Lymphs (Absolute)	3.0	
Monocytes (Absolute)	0.4	Monocytes (Absolute)	0.8	
Eos (Absolute)	0.2	Eos (Absolute)	0.2	
Baso (Absolute)	0.0	Baso (Absolute)	0.0	
Immature Granulocytes	0	Immature Granulocytes	0	
Immature Grans (Abs)	0.0			

Notice how the white blood cells increase as well as the platelets. The body is desperately trying to correct the massive influx of pathogens and toxins, but as you can see, it's failing to correct this imbalance. This "kill" caused this individual to have worsened arthritis and pain, which only added to their autoimmune condition.

You may wonder if it's possible to correct a CD4:CD8 ratio and thus stop autoimmune reactions without killing Lyme.

More simply, you may think your Lyme is causing poor immune function, so how can you restore immune function without killing Lyme?

If this is what you think, you haven't been paying attention.

Let's show how we boost and regulate your body's immunity without ever killing Lyme.

Before Treatment

CD4/CD8 Ratio Profile			
Absolute CD 4 Helper	417	/uL	359 - 1519
% CD 4 Pos. Lymph.	52.1	%	30.8 - 58.5
Abs. CD 8 Suppressor	208	/uL	109 - 897
% CD 8 Pos. Lymph.	26.0	%	12.0 - 35.5
CD4/CD8 Ratio	2.00		0.92 - 3.72

After 4 Weeks of Treatment

TESTS	RESULT	FLAG	UNITS	REFERENCE INTERVAL
CD4/CD8 Ratio Profile				
Absolute CD 4 Helper	774		/uL	359 - 1519
% CD 4 Pos. Lymph.	51.6		%	30.8 - 58.5
Abs. CD 8 Suppressor	422		/uL	109 - 897
% CD 8 Pos. Lymph.	28.1		%	12.0 - 35.5
CD4/CD8 Ratio	1.84			0.92 - 3.72

In terms of the CD4:CD8 absolute levels, a crucial value in representing immune function, this individual's immune function nearly doubled and was almost completely restored in just five weeks of our treatment, and yes, without ever killing this individual's Lyme. The person started with CD4 cells of 417/uL and CD8 cells of 208/uL (a good CD4:CD8 ratio) and after five short weeks jumped to 774 and 422 cells/uL (still a good ratio), respectively.

You may think (and be defensive) and say that this only one person, though. That can't happen multiple times without ever killing Lyme, right?

Well, here is another individual. This time, you can see how the ratio is 1.16 to begin with and is well on its way to regulating at 1.75 in just five weeks of treatment. If other issues are addressed, and with a great CD4:CD8 ratio, immune function can be restored quickly and stay balanced in the long term.

Before Treatment

TESTS	RESULT	FLAG	UNITS	REFERENCE INTERVAL
CD4/CD8 Ratio Profile				
Absolute CD 4 Helper	878		/uL	359 - 1519
% CD 4 Pos. Lymph.	46.2		%	30.8 - 58.5
Abs. CD 8 Suppressor	756		/uL	109 - 897
% CD 8 Pos. Lymph.	39.8	High	%	12.0 - 35.5
CD4/CD8 Ratio	1.16			0.92 - 3.72

After 5 Week of Treatment

TESTS	RESULT	FLAG	UNITS	REFERENCE INTERVAL
CD4/CD8 Ratio Profile				
Absolute CD 4 Helper	888		/uL	359 - 1519
% CD 4 Pos. Lymph.	55.5		%	30.8 - 58.5
Abs. CD 8 Suppressor	569		/uL	109 - 897
% CD 8 Pos. Lymph.	31.8		%	12.0 - 35.5
CD4/CD8 Ratio	1.75			0.92 - 3.72

It's much harder to correct the actual ratio than to merely boost immune function, especially when the ratio is below 2.0 (suppressive autoimmunity). Suppressive autoimmune ratios are seen in individuals with HIV and schizophrenia, among other conditions; thus, they shouldn't be taken lightly. If you think this massive disruption in immune function is from Lyme, you're kidding yourself.

Simply said, finding and stopping autoimmune reactions is one step, but healing the damage they've caused is another. Both are necessary in restoring immune function. Killing Lyme causes autoimmune symptoms to worsen and damage to increase.

One of the more recent bandwagons in terms of autoimmunity is the thyroid. Many physicians are testing thyroid values like TSH, free T3, free T4, TPO antibodies, and so on. Many fail to understand that if you have autoimmunity against your thyroid (attacking the thyroid), you have autoimmunity everywhere, including the brain. The only way to verify this condition is by testing. Thyroid is only one hormone, and TPO antibodies are only one immune value. You must run numerous hormones and numerous immune values to determine the extent of deficiency. I see a multitude of individuals arriving at my center convinced they have autoimmunity against their thyroids. We test an extensive immune and hormonal panel, with the usual results concluding almost every hormone and immune value is disrupted, which points toward autoimmunity. The thyroid isn't the whole picture, as you need more data. This concept shows up again when dealing with the gut because of the contrast between a true nutritional deficiency and overall malabsorption. You need extensive data from testing to truly understand each individual's needs for recovery from his or her health issues.

Simply said, thyroid autoimmunity, such as Graves' disease and Hashimoto's disease, points to a larger issue of body-wide autoimmunity. Moreover, thyroid is only one hormone, which never shows you the entire picture.

There are numerous other topics worth discussing in this section, but I want to touch on the vagus nerve, as it plays an enormous role in immune health (in terms of cytokine signaling, the inflammatory reflex, etc.), GI health (innervating more than half the GI system), and the cardiovascular system (innervating the heart). It also exemplifies how one component is capable of interacting with many different bodily systems (99, 100). The vagus nerve is one of the cranial nerves, which means it starts in the brain, and it projects significantly farther than any other cranial nerve, all the way down deep into the GI system. By calming the brain, you calm the vagus nerve. Noradrenaline and adrenaline (norepinephrine and epinephrine, respectively) play a significant role in the brain (as neurotransmitters) and in the heart as well. By calming excitatory chemicals, we're able to help the vagus nerve regulate the heart. We've seen individuals with arrhythmias, elevated heart rates, and dysfunction in blood pressure normalize merely by the brain being calmed. There's no doubt that calming the brain also affects the vagus nerve and the role it plays in the heart. By understanding your symptoms, we develop a functional neurology program that activates the vagus nerve. For example, singing loudly and gargling water are simple ways to activate the vagus nerve because they cause the uvula to move. This, when combined with our proprietary therapy, could potentially help with GI, immune, and cardiovascular symptoms. We assist in regulating the vagus nerve by analyzing and addressing your immune and inflammatory markers. Just this one nerve overlaps with the brain, the immune system, inflammatory cascades, the GI system, the cardiovascular system, and more. In addition, we use five to seven different tools when regulating the function of the vagus nerve.

Do you see how one component can basically span the entire body?

Do you see why you need these tools to address just that one component?

Do you see how everything is interconnected?

You must understand and use these tools to heal a multifaceted disease like Lyme.

Do you still think you should kill Lyme and disrupt the vagus nerve even more?

Simply said, the vagus nerve is an illustration of how your symptoms aren't separate from one another and how just this one component spans across four or more brain and bodily systems.

OK, that's your brief crash course in basic immune function and autoimmunity, but you mustn't forget that many prescription medications, which fall into the category of toxins, also cause autoimmunity.

Inflammation

Inflammation, as with disruptions in blood flow, occurs in every chronic disease, including Lyme. Inflammation must be addressed to achieve long-term healing. I'd say the top three contributors to autoimmunity are also the top three contributors to inflammation. Proper immune function and inflammation go hand in hand, so it's a good thing you already read that chapter. Most times, inflammation is the result of compromised immunity and blood flow. If you're constantly attacking yourself with dysregulated immune signaling, your body reacts by changing temperature, sending pain signals, swelling/puffing, and more; this is inflammation.

In terms of testing, a great indication of inflammation is C-reactive protein, or CRP. It increases because of immune activation. Therefore, if it's high, you have increased immune activation, and you likely have an increase in toxic load. This value also elevates when you break biofilms. (No surprise there.) Let's look at what happens when you stir up infections and toxic loads too quickly.

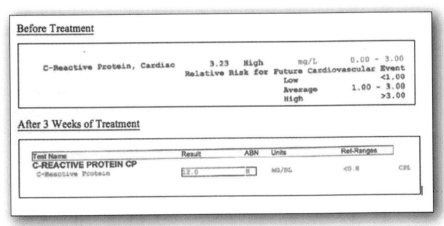

You can see how the value went from 3.23 to 12.0 mg/L; that's an increase of more than 271 percent!

We see countless individuals who experience a whole bunch of "itises" - tonsillitis, sinusitis, gastritis, arthritis, tendonitis, rhinitis - and they rarely happen once. Most of the time, inflammatory infections show up time and time again, almost like clockwork. At times, they appear unrelated, and they sometimes occurred when you were a child or teenager.

What's the treatment used most often for infections?

Antibiotics.

Not only are early infections, frequent infections, and inflammation signs of underlying issues, but the standard treatment for these conditions fails to address this underlying cause. Plus, the overuse of antibiotics has detrimental effects on your brain, immune system, and GI health.

Simply said, inflammation is like autoimmunity because it has many of the same contributory factors. Most people agree inflammation is one symptom that occurs with great severity in chronic Lyme patients.

Chronic Lyme individuals usually have high amounts of inflammation in their bodies. Yet much of the time, we see individuals with Lyme who are testing with low inflammation because their brains and bodies are slowly shutting down. Immune and brain signaling are compromised, causing an inability to initiate inflammatory reactions. This doesn't mean their inflammation is non-existent; it means their bodies' ability to communicate, initiate, and regulate inflammation is nonexistent. Moreover, if you decide to kill Lyme, either you will cause your current inflammation to worsen, which will cause your symptoms to worsen, or you will jump-start the inflammatory process, which has been shut down for some time. This causes years of unprocessed inflammation to suddenly come to the surface. This is yet another reason why you shouldn't kill your Lyme, just in case I haven't given you enough reasons already.

Environmental/Industrial Toxicity

I've talked about toxicity, and now it's time to expand my thoughts and beliefs. Let me start by telling you what I mean by environmental and industrial toxins. I'll review what I've mentioned in previous sections. Toxins can be divided into two categories: toxins that dissolve in fat and toxins that dissolve in water (fat-soluble and water-soluble toxins, respectively). We're not deeply concerned with water-soluble toxins, because they dissolve into urine and are flushed out much more easily. Fat-soluble toxins—or fatty toxins, as I call them—are much more difficult to eradicate. These are the toxins I refer to when I talk about toxicity, whether environmental or industrial. Most times, toxins are so small that they go unrecognized by your own immune system, causing harmful effects before your brain and body are aware of any problems. Therefore, we test your genetics to determine your susceptibility to fatty toxins. If you possess the HLA gene and are susceptible to fatty toxins, you move out fatty toxins exponentially more slowly than people without this gene. To make matters even worse, numerous Lyme individuals possess this gene, and we've found that more than 93 percent of people with Lyme at our center have this gene; the national average is between 25 and 30 percent. Both environmental and industrial sources produce fatty toxins, causing an alarming threat to your brain and body; however, in addition to having toxins, the immune system of a person suffering from Lyme is always somewhat dysfunctional. The HLA gene causes you to eliminate toxins hundreds of times more slowly than individuals without the gene, so elimination is undoubtedly even slower among Lyme individuals.

Simply said, when I'm talking about environmental and industrial toxins, I'm referring mainly to fatty toxins for multiple reasons. Fatty toxins are most commonly encountered and cause an ever-growing list of damages to Lyme individuals, especially those with dangerous genetic risk factors.

Fatty toxins aren't the only type of toxin, but they're the most common toxins that our tests reveal in Lyme individuals. The reason I stress fatty toxins so often is their potency, which has debilitating effects in Lyme individuals.

Why Do Fatty Toxins Pose Such a Threat to Us?

Fatty toxins pose a threat to us because they attack fatty things in our bodies. What is fat in the body?

- Your brain is about 60 percent fat.
- Your myelin sheaths are 80 percent fat. (These sheaths for neurons are responsible for fast communication in the brain.)
- Your cells' gatekeeper, the cell membrane, is a fatty bilayer.
- You have fat cells and fat tissues.

Fatty toxins enter your fat cells, eliciting immune signals (cytokines) that disrupt blood vessels, affecting circulation (increased clotting factors) and oxygenation (reduced VEGF), while increasing inflammation and immune symptoms (increased MMP-9, TNF-alpha, IL-1B, C3a, and C4a). This leads to a multitude of symptoms, including increased susceptibility to any immune disturbance, including food allergies. They also send different signals (cytokines and increased leptin) that make their way to the brain (hypothalamus), causing a reduced output of hormones (MSH, then ACTH, ADH, melatonin, and sex hormones), which leads to symptoms such as sleep issues, chronic pain, frequent urination, GI issues, prolonged illness, and decreased libido and reproductive output (101). Fatty toxins travel to the brain, where they destroy the barrier to the brain (the astrocytes of the blood-brain barrier), then make their way to brain cells (neurons), which they destroy almost on contact (24). They attack proteins in the myelin sheath, which is responsible for the way the brain communicates electrically. This leads to a multitude of issues, such as brain fog; memory problems; and balance, motor, and coordination problems, as well as neurodegenerative diseases. Sometimes damage to the myelin sheath from fatty toxins causes white spots that appear on MRIs, showing destruction of the brain. Fatty toxins disrupt the cell membrane, affecting cell structure, communication, and mobility, leading to a medley of symptoms.

Why? Because fatty toxins attack fatty things in your body. These are some types of damage that occur in your brain and body, but this is by no means the full extent of fatty toxins' possible devastation.

Simply said, fatty toxins damage fatty things in your body. Your brain is approximately 60 percent fat, the myelin sheath in your brain is approximately 80 percent fat, and your cells' gatekeeper is a fatty bilayer. In addition you have fat cells and fat tissues. This makes your brain and body highly susceptible to fatty toxins, especially if you possess the HLA gene.

Why Do You Emphasize Mold Toxicity?

I emphasize mold toxicity because it is fully capable of the destruction I just mentioned; however, it goes much further than that. The most common fatty toxin we see is mold toxins (mycotoxins). Yeah, yeah, mold is bad, we know, but you don't realize how much damage mold toxicity can cause. Many common molds produce toxins that become airborne and pose great threats to everyone. Many know not to eat white, fuzzy strawberries or bluish-black bread because there's mold on them. However, did you know that breathing in the toxins that mold produces is worse than ingesting the actual mold (102)? Did you know that mold toxins can also enter through your skin and that they've been mentioned and implicated in biological warfare (111)? There's a debate about whether mold toxins can affect you only if they're ingested. To be honest, this is laughable. This claim usually comes from closed-minded individuals (and physicians) who haven't done any research and don't have much expertise in chronic disease, but I'll leave you with this comment: if mold toxins (trichothecene specifically, the black mold toxin) have been implicated in biological warfare (yellow rain in Southeast Asia), warfare that involves airborne exposure mechanisms to inflict widespread death or debilitating symptoms, isn't that enough to prove it's harmful to breathe in mycotoxins? Trichothecene is four hundred times more potent than mustard gas in producing skin lesions (111). Oh, and "with larger doses in humans, aerosolized trichothecenes may produce death within minutes to hours…trichothecene mycotoxins have an excellent potential for weaponization" (111). But hey, I'm sure you're right, and mold toxins don't cause much harm; they surely don't cause much effect if breathed in or absorbed through the skin.

As I said, laughable.

Anyway, you'll get symptoms from airborne, skin, and ingestion exposure, but airborne mold toxins are the most common, the most prevalent, and the most detrimental. It's imperative we understand that breathable toxins are more dangerous, because our exposure to airborne mycotoxins is much higher than our exposure to ingestible mycotoxins.

The NIH estimates that between 30 and 50 percent of homes have poor air quality due to mold toxins; this is also known as sick building syndrome (24). Recent studies also show we spend up to 90 percent of our time indoors (18). With home builders' recent attempts to save money and become more and more energy efficient, they have used plant-based drywall (mold's food source), and many buildings have been built to be airtight (controlled breeding conditions for mold). This makes mold a serious threat to all of us, especially if you possess the HLA gene, because your body can't recognize and move the toxins out of your system. My strong emphasis on mold is based on our lifestyles and our environment as human beings, because mold is the most abundant environmental toxin all of us encounter. Mold toxins, as well as other fatty toxins, are quite simple to remove; we do it in a matter of a few weeks. Below is an example of an individual who tried to get rid of trichothecene toxins multiple times prior to arriving at our center, with no success (as documented on the test). After just four weeks of our treatment, his trichothecene (the most potent of all mold toxins) dropped from 1.58 parts per billion (ppb) (eight times the "accepted" rate) to 0.26 ppb, a negligible amount.

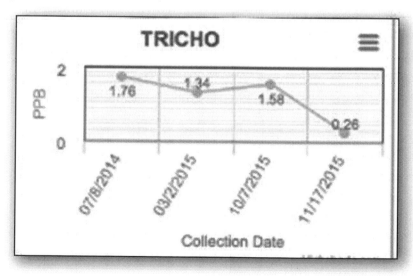

Here is another example of an individual who spent a lot of time in their room suffering from debilitating fatigue, headaches, and insomnia, all of which can be caused by elevated mold toxins.

See how the trichothecene dropped from 2.11 ppb (over ten times the "accepted" rate) to 0.16 ppb (which is next to nothing and considered negative) in just four weeks of treatment. We did a follow-up test three months later (with no additional treatment except for supplements) to ensure the toxic load remained low, and it decreased even further to 0.05 ppb, showing that this individual is now fully capable of eliminating these toxins without continuous care.

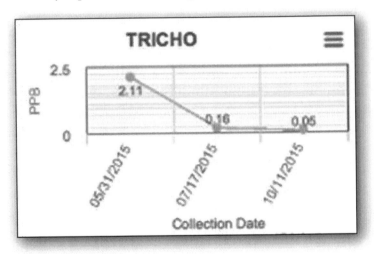

Simply said, mold toxins are the most common fatty toxins present in individuals, especially individuals suffering from Lyme disease, and it's absolutely crucial to eradicate toxins to ensure both short term and long term healing.

There is some argument regarding the validity of mold tests in general, since overall groups and not individual toxins are tested. Some argue that the T-2 toxin is not as common, yet many of the studies on the damages of mold involve T-2. I am completely aware of these arguments, and I do not reject them. What I reject is the laughable notion that mold can't cause problems and that it rarely plays a role; that is what is ridiculous. However, just as with everything, we don't hang our hat on only one issue, and that includes mold toxicity. I'm going to continue outlining the potential damage and what you need to know about toxicity; what I want you to keep in mind is that all environmental/industrial toxicity, including mold toxicity, can and usually does play a role in all chronic diseases, including Lyme; however, as all diseases are multifaceted, it is not the only piece.

What Are These Toxins, and What Are They Capable of Harming?

In general, when speaking of toxins, I'm referring mainly to fatty toxins, but this doesn't exclude many common industrial toxins listed below. Let me start off by answering some questions you may have.

What's the difference between environmental and industrial toxins?

What are some examples of those toxins?

What are they capable of harming?

Environmental toxins are naturally occurring toxins, while industrial toxins are basically man-made toxins. Fatty toxins are the most common, but as I said, there are numerous other toxins that are just as, or even more, dangerous. As mentioned, the major difference is frequency of exposure. I talk about fatty toxins more often because they appear most frequently in Lyme individuals, but this doesn't change the fact that all toxins need to be addressed and removed. Let me give you some examples.

- Mold toxins (mycotoxins) - environmental fatty toxins
- Benzene (smoke, fires - used to make gasoline, plastics, resins, pesticides, preservatives, etc.) - environmental and industrial fatty toxins
- Toluene (paints, thinners, gasoline, shoe polish, glues) - environmental and industrial fatty toxins
- Formaldehyde (adhesives, bonding agents, pressed wood [hardwood floors], foam insulation, synthetic clothing fibers, personal and cosmetic products) - environmental and industrial fatty toxins
- Phthalates - industrial toxins
- PVC (polyvinyl chloride) - industrial toxin
- Heavy metals - environmental and industrial toxins
- Ammonia - environmental and industrial toxin

- Pesticides - industrial toxins (can be fatty)
- Many preservatives - industrial toxins (can be fatty)

Many toxins come in multiple forms. For example, you've heard of benzoic acid, which is a common preservative in cosmetics, foods, and beverages. Benzoic acid reacts with vitamin C to make benzene, and since our bodies always have vitamin C on hand, benzoic acid is basically benzene. Numerous sodas, including many orange-flavored sodas, contain both benzoic acid and vitamin C. This causes a reaction inside the bottle before you drink it; it makes benzene. The FDA conducted its own study showing many sodas exceeding the 5 ppb allowable limit, with one brand exceeding this maximum limit by fifteen times (103). Moreover, toluene converts to methylhippuric acid (MHA). When both MHA and benzoic acid are present, it becomes more difficult to get rid of both toxins than it is if only one is present.

Exposure to toxins is one thing, but you must understand the damage they do to the brain and body. I've mentioned a few toxins below, but in large part, these are categories, as many chemicals change form as they're broken down in your body into metabolites. They come in many shapes and sizes, and sometimes metabolites are more dangerous, sometimes less; regardless, you must remove them. We do just that. Here are some detrimental effects that have been linked to some of the most common toxins:

Mold toxins

- Stop your cells from replicating (stop DNA/RNA synthesis, irreversibly bind to large subunit of ribosomes) (21)
- Inhibit protein synthesis (111)
- Cause lipid peroxidation (damage to anything containing lipids [fats], as I've stated) to the liver, spleen, kidneys, and thymus
- Cause damage to bone marrow with one dose of T-2 (trichothecene, black mold toxin) (111)
- Inhibit mitochondria synthesis (111)
- Destroy brain cells (neurons) (24)

- Destroy the barrier between the body and the brain (blood-brain barrier—astrocytes) (24)
- Destroy the myelin sheath (24, 104)
- Disrupt the cells' gatekeeper (cell membrane) (107)
- Destroy brain endothelial cells (24, 104)
- Cause pituitary tumors (adenomas) (105)
- Are equivalent to minor traumatic brain injury (24)
- Cause short-term memory loss and disorientation (24, 106)
- Cause disruptions in balance and coordination (106)
- Cause ADHD and short-term memory issues (106)
- Cause stress to the brain and body (oxidative stress) (23)
- Decrease energy output (disrupt mitochondria) (21, 108)
- Destroy cartilage cells (chondrocytes) (22) - joint pain, chronic pain
- Destroy heart cells (cardiomyocytes) (20) - arrhythmias, high blood pressure
- Disrupt gut lining and can cause gut lining necrosis (death) (109) - malabsorption, autoimmunity
- Disrupt immunity and cause inflammation (TNF-alpha, many interleukins and cytokines) (19, 110) - susceptibility to Lyme and other infections
- Suppress reproductive organ and hormonal function - (111)
- Can cause cancers (113)
- Lower oxygen delivery - lower VEGF (17)
- Contribute to autoimmunity, leaky gut, and gluten sensitivity (17)
- Elevate proinflammatory cytokines (17)
- Cause central and peripheral neuropathies (114)
- Cause chronic fatigue syndrome (114)
- Cause liver disease and elevated liver enzymes (112)
- Cause asthma and breathing issues (24, 113)

Benzene

- Causes chromosomal and mitotic spindle damage (115)
- Causes liver damage (115)
- Causes kidney damage (115)

- Causes hormonal disruption (116)
- Causes oxidative stress (damage) (117)
- Can cause cancer (117)

Toluene

- Causes reproductive and developmental issues (118)

Heavy metals

- Can cause cancer (119)
- Cause heart issues (119)
- Cause lung issues (119)
- Cause liver issues (119)
- Cause kidney issues (119)
- Cause GI issues (119)

To those who were laughed at or mocked by their physicians for bringing up mold as a potential cause of your symptoms, I am sorry. For those who think mold is a joke, please join the twenty-first century. Toxins affect multiple brain and bodily systems, and although I don't mean to scare you, mold toxicity must be taken seriously. Hopefully, this was illuminating. Some of the types of damage that have been documented explain some of your symptoms quite well. We've proven toxicity plays a significantly larger role in your symptoms than does Lyme disease itself. Moreover, mold toxins have an incredible effect on the immune system while causing immune suppression. Often, a compromised immune system allows Lyme and other coinfections into your system to develop in the first place!

Simply said, the detrimental effects of fatty toxins are quite vast. We've proven that at times toxicity explains your Lyme symptoms more than Lyme itself does. I hope you're beginning to understand the necessity for a multitool approach.

These effects are not to be taken lightly; you must take toxicity seriously and address it quickly.

How Do You Address Toxicity Properly?

You surely don't go around breaching biofilms to rid toxins, as can be seen below.

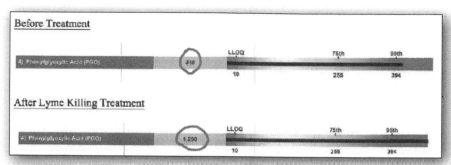

This harmful toxin (PGO, usually found in plastics) was already extremely elevated at 410 before this individual started treatment at another clinic. After treatment, it jumped off the charts to 1,290. That's an increase of more than 214 percent.

This is yet another example of the many drawbacks of therapies aimed at killing Lyme and breaching biofilms. OK, now back to the process of properly addressing toxicity.

First, you test for toxins. You remove many of them with simple mechanisms that I've researched and tested time and time again, but we want to be precise, and that requires testing.

Second, you must understand what elevated levels of a certain toxin mean. Where could the toxicity be coming from? What brain or body system will be affected most? For example, mold toxins usually come from your home or your work. Quite differently, ammonia is most often associated with pathogenic bacteria in the gut (Helicobacter pylori, or H. pylori, produces ammonia to help it survive in your gut) and an excess breakdown of proteins. Thus, we remove both toxins; however, if we don't know where the toxicity is coming from, then it doesn't make much of a difference.

Third, elevated level is a relative term. Certain toxins are much more potent than others, even within their own categories. For example, mycotoxins comprise mainly aflatoxin, ochratoxin, and trichothecene, which are produced by many different mold species. Trichothecene is five times more potent than aflatoxin and ten times more potent than ochratoxin. So, a level of, let's say, three parts per billion of aflatoxin, ochratoxin, and trichothecene would be considered elevated for each of these three toxins, yet trichothecene is much more dangerous because of its potency relative to the other two toxins. Elevation is relative, and some toxins are more common and more dangerous than others.

Fourth, you must understand how to remove toxins. When you pinpoint where the toxins are coming from, you can successfully remove them. You're on the right path, but you're not done yet.

Fifth, you need to know how to quickly remove toxins. If you move too fast, you get dramatic immune activation and an increase of symptoms like die-off. If you move too slowly, treatment lasts for months, even years, which isn't necessary. Speed is also a crucial step in toxicity removal.

The sixth and probably most overlooked step in treating mold toxicity is that you must fix the damage caused by the toxins. Please read the list above again. The potency of toxins can be brutal, but merely removing the toxins is not enough for Lyme individuals.

But what happens when you breach the biofilm?

I've stated numerous times that toxins are located within the biofilm; therefore, if you breach the biofilm in an attempt to kill Lyme, your toxic load will escalate. Below, you can see four toxins that were tested on this individual prior to treatment. These toxins are 2-hydroxyisobutyric acid (parent toxin is MTBE), monoethylphthalate (parent toxins are diethylphthalates), 2-3-4 methylhippuric acid (parent toxin is xylene), and phenylglyoxylic acid (parent toxins are styrene and ethylbenzene). These toxins are found in gasoline/contaminated groundwater, pharmaceuticals/beauty products, paints/pesticides, and plastics/pollution, respectively. The point is that these are industrial toxins that were all present in relatively low amounts prior to Lyme treatment. You can see below the following values for each of these toxins: 3,837 (~50th percentile) for MTBE, 5.7 (~5th percentile) for diethylphthlates, 56 (~10th percentile) for xylene, and 151 (~40th percentile) for styrene/ethylbenzene. The units for all these values are in ug/g creatinine.

Before Treatment

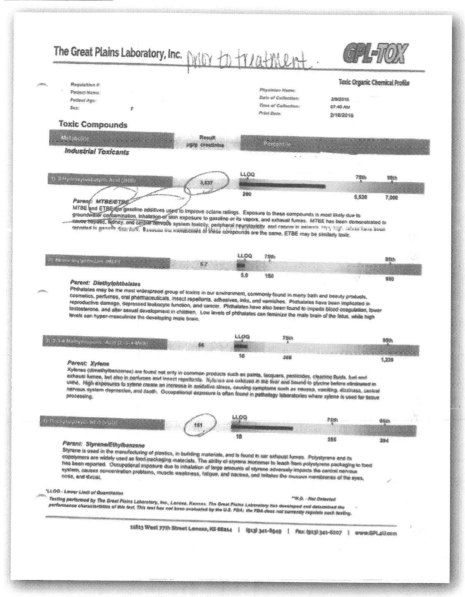

Now, notice how these same toxins were elevated after this individual underwent just one week of treatment for Lyme at another clinic!

After 1 Week of Lyme "Kill" Treatment

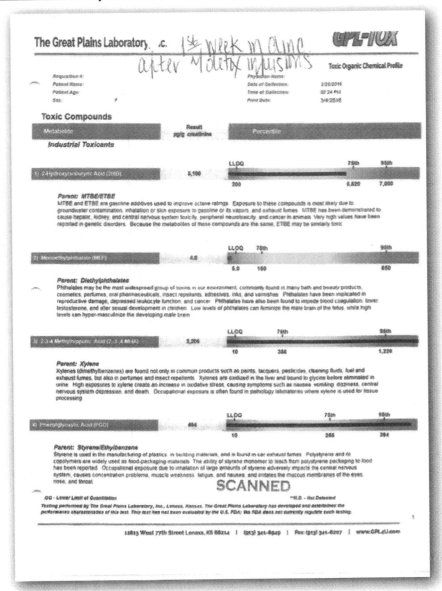

MTBE jumped to about the 70th percentile at 5,190, while the toxins xylene and styrene/ethylbenzene jumped off the charts into the 99th percentile at 2,206, and 464, respectively (all in units of ug/g creatinine). Fortunately, in a rare instance, the diphthlalates remained relatively unchanged. MTBE increased by 35 percent while stylene/ethylbenzene and xylene increased by a whopping 207 percent and 3,840 percent, respectively. Imagine the damage that months or even years of this type of treatment could do to one's brain and body.

This increase in toxins leads to more inflammation, brain imbalance, issues with blood flow, and more. Not only did this increase in toxins show up in additional testing, but this individual experienced more brain fog, more seizure-like activity, and more depression. You should be beginning to realize why you should not kill Lyme.

Moreover, most of these toxins are processed in the liver. During Lyme treatments, your physician controls the speed at which you are killing Lyme; this leads to uncontrolled breaches of the biofilm and uncontrollable increases in toxins from the biofilm. This puts enormous stress on the liver, which is indicated in a liver enzyme blood test. Liver enzymes appear elevated in the blood when there's damage occurring to the liver. You can see this below.

Before Treatment		
AST	20	10-30 U/L
ALT	13	6-29 U/L
After Lyme Killing Treatment		
AST	76 H	10-30 U/L
ALT	179 H	6-29 U/L

I believe these tests speak for themselves, but you see the enzymes AST and ALT began at 20 U/L and 13 U/L, respectively, and jumped to 76 U/L and 179 U/L, respectively, upon Lyme treatment. That's an increase of 280 percent in AST and 1,277 percent in ALT! AST is found in both the liver and the muscle, but ALT is found almost exclusively in the liver. These toxins are no joke, and breaching the biofilm only further contributes to their burden in the brain and body. This is the reason toxins are linked to liver damage and even cancer.

Simply said, addressing, removing, and healing the damage that fatty toxins pose is a multistep, precise process. Each step is crucial. Trying to kill Lyme only contributes to your toxic load and decreases your chances of getting better.

A Touch More on Toxicity and Autoimmunity, and Yes, Some More Science

Toxicity is a major contributor to autoimmunity and inflammation, but black mold toxins (trichothecene) cause so much inflammation and immune activation they provoke disturbances in gall bladder activity, therefore increasing the likelihood of the removal of the gall bladder in many individuals. Since toxicity plays such a large role in immune dysfunction, it comes as no surprise that your spleen and red blood cells are dramatically affected by toxicity. Many toxins cause stress in your cells, especially your red blood cells, the cells that carry oxygen to your brain and body. Your red blood cells are supposed to be perfectly round discs with a smooth, circular cell membrane. Toxins cause the outer layer, the cell membrane (the gatekeeper), to become imprecisely jagged, affecting cell structure and cell function. Your spleen monitors your red blood cells, ensuring there's no funny business going on, and when the life span of a red blood cell is over, the spleen sends signals for it to be removed and recycled. If your spleen recognizes jagged-edged red blood cells, it removes them prematurely. We see many individuals with low blood flow, but sometimes it's caused by the spleen's perception of these supposed deformed cells, and their untimely disposal lowers the number of red blood cells available. On top of that, toxins cause lower oxygen delivery by lowering VEGF, further contributing to poor blood flow (perfusion). This is one single mechanism by which toxins cause autoimmunity and low blood flow.

Another mechanism shows toxins binding to carrier molecules like albumin and subsequently binding to your own tissues, causing your immune system to go haywire, resulting in autoimmunity. Mold toxins as well as many other industrial and environmental toxins, such as formaldehyde, benzene, toluene, many anhydrides, ethylenes, and even medications, are among the most potent in the mechanism of autoimmunity. The bottom line is you must remove toxins from your brain and body

The most likely mechanism of autoimmunity by fatty-toxin toxicity is through excess immune activation. Immune signalers just go wild and skyrocket when they see toxins, especially if you possess the HLA gene. As various markers, such as matrix metallopeptidase 9 (MMP-9), begin to elevate and immune signalers cause a cascade of events to occur (cytokines provoke interleukins), nasty stuff begins to happen. Eventually the "nukes" of the immune system become activated, including tumor necrosis factor alpha, or TNF-alpha, whose elevation has been indicated in almost every autoimmune condition and which is the target of the number one immune-suppressing pharmaceutical drug, Humira˚. MMP-9 can cross the blood brain barrier and elicit autoimmunity in the brain as well as in the body. We've also seen many individuals who have antibodies against their myelin sheaths from fatty toxin toxicity; that's autoimmunity against your brain's electrical-conducting system, by the way. If MMP-9, cytokines, and interleukins remain elevated, so do the resulting immune responses. If left unchecked, this quickly turns into autoimmunity. Therefore, many individuals with this gene stay sick much longer; over time autoimmunity becomes so bad you no longer get sick in the traditional sense. These same toxins also cause a leaky gut, further contributing to autoimmunity. Yes, foods play a significant role, but toxins cannot be overlooked. Did you know toxicity enhances the detrimental effects of gliadin, the protein fragment from gluten? This further contributes to gluten sensitivity.

Simply said, if left unchecked in your system, toxins cause autoimmunity and great damage to your red blood cells.

I've Tried Removing Toxins, but I've Been Unsuccessful

There are many essential steps that must be taken to properly address toxicity, and two ways physicians fail at alleviating the burden of toxicity are by not understanding pathways to get rid of toxins and by not knowing how to fix the damage they've caused. Many prefer methods that grab toxins - what I like to call grabbers, like zeolite, charcoal, red clay, and more - but this is only one mechanism and works only for a certain category of toxins. Physicians are still using cholestyramine to remove mold toxins, as if the year weren't 2016. My deepest thanks go to Dr. Shoemaker for all his contributions, but it's been twelve years; come on, people. On top of that, you have physicians claiming all your problems are derived from mold in your nose and sinuses. Really? Complex, chronic, treatment-resistant diseases stemming from nasal biofilms? Plain and simple: localized and single faceted approaches are not going to give you the best chance to heal. Sometimes people think that if they have the HLA gene, toxins can never be removed, when in fact this is far from the truth; you just need the proper tools. Most toxins, especially fatty toxins, must be broken down into metabolites to reduce their potency to allow your body to eradicate them; grabbers prove to be mostly ineffective in this regard. As I've stated numerous times, you must access multiple tools even within one category of toxins. You can't have just a plain screwdriver; you must have a flathead and a Phillips head with multiple sizes and thicknesses of each. Sometimes you need a nail gun or power tool. It's great you have a Phillips head, but that won't screw in every nail and screw.

WHAT HAPPENS WHEN I LEAVE YOUR CENTER?

Many individuals leaving our center are concerned about how to keep harmful toxins at a manageable level, especially after reading and hearing about all the damaging effects they have. No one can be completely toxin-free. This doesn't mean you live your life in a protective bubble in fear. You can easily live your life in a way so that toxins no longer have a large effect. You must keep your radar on high alert. We educate you on the removal process and teach you what signs to look for so you can avoid future exposure; that's basically it. We take care of the rest; we remove the toxins and heal the damage they've caused, thus taking the burden of toxicity off your shoulders. Once this burden is removed, our education and tools keep you well once you return home.

Yes, we'll provide you with a long-term supplementation regimen that's been proven over the years to make sure your toxin load will remain low. However, there are easy changes you should begin to implement in your lifestyle. The easiest way to combat environmental toxins is by changing the environment itself. You beat toxins by excretion: by sweating, by urinating, and by defecating. You beat toxins by being outside in the sunlight, away from pollution. You beat toxins by exercising or using saunas or steam rooms or peat baths to sweat the toxins out. You beat toxins by consuming the proper amount of water. This, along with our treatment, our education, and our long-term care, will lift this burden from your shoulders forever.

Simply said, once we've properly removed and healed the damage caused by fatty toxins, we educate you with knowledge that keeps you healthy. You must keep your radar on high alert for toxins, but you should never, ever live in fear of them.

What to Eat and What Not to Eat

When individuals are suffering from various health issues, especially Lyme disease, the first place they go to research is the Internet. They're searching for possible answers and treatment options, seeking opportunities to take charge of their own health. One of the most common answers to explore is the possibility that foods are causing many of their symptoms. There's no question: the answers to many health issues can be found in the foods we eat. Yes, there are many other contributory factors, but if you don't believe the food you eat plays a tremendous role in your health, you're struggling with reality. My goal in writing this book is to provide my thoughts backed with sound science to help chronic Lyme individuals understand their disease, to help them realize there's a better way. I would estimate that more than 95 percent of individuals who come to our center have already made beneficial dietary choices. With chronically ill individuals, the problem is that common lifestyle choices, such as a good diet and good food choices, aren't sufficient to provide enough symptom relief to allow healing. The severity of your disease can sometimes dictate the amount of relief you'll find in certain treatment options—hence, my belief in attacking disease from all different angles. However, it doesn't change the fact that positive dietary choices are a crucial step in the healing process.

In the next few paragraphs, I'll outline some brief facts about a few dietary choices I believe most individuals suffering from chronic Lyme should abide by. I could write an entire book on diet, food, pesticides, GMOs, and the types of diets I've seen individuals at our center using, but you can find most of this information that I've pieced together on the Internet and from others. Please don't misinterpret my intention as not emphasizing food and diet; this couldn't be further from the truth. It's just not the focus of this book because, quite frankly, the majority of individuals have already eliminated some of the most symptom-provoking foods, which are most commonly known as food allergens.

Simply said, a good diet and the elimination of symptom-provoking foods play a tremendous role in symptom reduction and are two of the most crucial steps in healing from any chronic disease.

What Are Some Symptom-Provoking Foods?

Individuals frequently ask about diet, with the most common question being "What's the number one thing I should avoid?" To be honest, my answer is gluten; however, everyone is different. Ranking food allergies wouldn't be fair, as many of you experience different symptoms and symptom severity from different foods. So whether it's gluten, dairy, grains, legumes, nightshades, corn, soy, rice, or others, the truth is that all of them can (and have been documented to) cause serious symptoms in many bodily systems, including the brain. Many may be familiar with foods causing gut (GI) symptoms, such as diarrhea, indigestion, and nausea, but it may come as a surprise that these foods have been linked to serious autoimmune and neurological complications, such as ADHD, autism, Alzheimer's, anxiety, bipolar disease, brain lesions, Crohn's, cognitive dysfunction, depression, migraines, motor and coordination dysfunction, multiple sclerosis, schizophrenia, seizures, and many more.

How is it possible that food could contribute to these conditions?

Foods—more specifically, food allergens or symptom-provoking foods—cause inflammation, immune and blood-flow dysfunction, and much more. The truth is that every disease, especially chronic diseases like Lyme, lead to these very conditions: inflammation and immune and blood-flow dysfunction. (Yes, there are additional conditions, and yes, I will discuss them also.) In an ideal world, I'd rather our individuals ask us what they should gravitate toward, not away from. This mentality, again, shows the fear that medicine has created in individuals, but that's for another day.

In this section, I'll show the science and studies behind these claims as well as some of the mechanisms by which they occur. It's difficult to determine which food allergen is the most serious for each person, but gluten is the most common and probably one of the worst. Corn, rice, and wheat are the most consumed grains in the world; they are used to make various foods such as baked goods, pastas, noodles, couscous, and breads. A gluten-free diet is used primarily to treat celiac disease (complete gluten intolerance), but it's growing in popularity among those who are gluten sensitive (nonceliac gluten sensitive [NCGS]). A gluten-free diet consists of dietary choices that do not have the gluten protein, which is found in these foods along with barley and rye. Other foods, such as chicken broth, malt vinegar, and some salad dressings, can have gluten. There are also many hidden sources of gluten, such as processed meats and soy sauce. The reaction to gluten is a reaction to the protein fractions gliadin and glutenin, which cause a cascade of symptoms that usually starts in the gut; however, a growing body of research shows gluten's relationship to other immune and inflammatory markers (mast cells, basophils, and histamine) as well as autoimmunity and its resulting complications.

Simply said, gluten is linked to serious disorders, including neurological and neurodegenerative diseases. It's also been proven to play a tremendous role in autoimmunity and inflammation.

Do individuals feel better after they stop eating foods containing gluten? In my opinion, everyone who stops eating gluten will probably feel better; however, symptom improvement varies from individual to individual. As mentioned above, most individuals arriving at our clinic have already stopped eating gluten, but often this action hasn't provided much symptom relief. It's a necessary step regardless. The bottom line is if you're suffering from chronic Lyme or any other chronic disease, you should not eat gluten—period! It's just not worth it. The threat of contributing further to autoimmunity, inflammation, and the severity of your symptoms is too great.

Simply said, if you have Lyme or any other chronic disease, gluten should be eliminated from your diet.

The overall mechanism of many food allergies is similar, and I'll outline it in the next paragraph. (This is basically the same mechanism that I discussed in the section on the cons of antibiotics.) Food allergies usually operate by this similar overall mechanism, but they have their own intricacies as well. Gluten's intricate mechanism proves to be very detrimental to your brain. Quite honestly, even if you're not suffering from a chronic disease like Lyme, you shouldn't be eating gluten if you care about the longevity and quality of your brain. Here's why:

At Lifestyle Healing Institute, we take a snapshot of your brain and body by looking at multiple systems individually, then we analyze how these systems function together as a whole unit using objective biochemical testing. One of the systems we analyze is the gastrointestinal (GI) system, or the gut, to understand its overall functionality. People often say, "You are what you eat," but that's not the entire picture. One of my teachers said it best when he told us, "You are what you assimilate and what you do not eliminate." Basically, if you can't absorb and integrate what you eat (assimilate), your dietary choices don't mean that much. Also, if you can't get rid of the waste you accumulate (eliminate), you're storing more toxins and waste. If these pathways (and many more) aren't optimized, your GI system will suffer, and you'll more than likely have resulting symptoms.

One of the most common symptoms among our Lyme individuals is a poor gut. Some individuals we've treated have developed a poor gut over time (often through antibiotic overuse) and/or have at some point developed unresolved food allergies. Most individuals also arrive at our clinic with a medley of GI symptoms, including acid reflux, constipation, indigestion, diarrhea, bloating, and irritable bowel syndrome/disease. Much of the time, their overall absorption is vastly compromised, which manifests in many of the aforementioned symptoms. When your gut lining (tight junctions) becomes compromised, the propensity for some materials to begin to leak out into places they're not supposed to will increase. This is what's known as a leaky gut, or leaky gut syndrome, if you want fancy terminology. If you're constantly having an inflammatory, immune-based response to different foods, your beneficial bacteria become depleted, and your gut lining becomes more and more compromised, resulting in more leakage. This results in a less acidic gut pH and the inability to break down foods, as well as increases in inflammation. This means as you ingest and digest your food, some of it isn't fully digested, and these undigested food particles are leaking out of the GI system and into the bloodstream. Because food particles aren't supposed to be there, your immune system recognizes them as abnormal and tags them as foreign, which results in an attack against these foreign particles. This leads to an unwanted activation of your immune system, resulting in inflammation and autoimmunity, or the body attacking itself. You're now attacking your own blood, your own GI system, and your own body.

If that's not bad enough, eventually some of these foreign particles, and sometimes their accompanying abnormal immune cascades, make their way to the brain through the blood-brain barrier, causing even more damage by disrupting the integrity of brain regions and neurotransmitter systems. The symptoms of a leaky gut can be quite serious. If you're already prone to autoimmunity and/or inflammation from your genetics, environment, and so on, a leaky gut contributes to your existing symptoms. Although individuals exhibit a multitude of symptoms across numerous brain and bodily systems, I've yet to see an individual come through our doors without inflammation and/or autoimmunity.

Simply said, the overall mechanism of food allergies begins in the gut, but over time the resulting abnormal immune reactions make their way to the brain and bloodstream, resulting in immune and inflammatory cascades, which greatly contribute to your symptoms.

Up to this point, the overall mechanism of autoimmunity has been relatively the same for all food allergens or symptom-provoking foods. However, please note that each of these foods has additional ramifications, resulting in more specific autoimmunity. For gluten, this intricacy is quite damaging.

In the brain, you've got cells called Purkinje cells inside the cerebellum; they play an intricate role in the overall integrity of both the cerebellum and overall brain function. The cerebellum itself has a loop of communication among regions of the brain, and its integrity has an immense impact on overall brain function and cognition (120). The protein fractions of gluten look like Purkinje cells (a phenomenon known as molecular mimicry), which poses a problem for your immune system. Through a leaky gut, these protein fractions make their way to the brain. Your immune system has difficulty differentiating between your own Purkinje cells and these foreign particles, the gluten protein fragments. It then proceeds to produce antibodies to the foreign particles, telling your immune system to get rid of them; however, there's a problem. The striking similarity between gluten protein fragments and your own Purkinje cells makes it too difficult for your immune system to differentiate between them. The result is your immune system produces antibodies to your Purkinje cells, your own cerebellum, causing immune activation against your own brain, from resulting cross-reactive T cells. This is autoimmunity against your brain with results detrimental beyond explanation. This is the best mechanism to explain how gluten protein fragments can drastically damage the Purkinje cells in the cerebellum and thus overall brain function and cognition. Regardless of what mechanism you feel makes the most sense, the bottom line is that gluten has severe consequences for the Purkinje cells of the cerebellum (77). If the cerebellum is damaged, so are cognition and overall functionality of the entire brain (120). It's unnecessary to risk further damaging your brain and body when you're already experiencing such severe symptoms.

Dairy, soy, grains, legumes, and nightshades have their own intricacies as well, but in the end, they usually involve some sort of antibody production against a material that's in the wrong place (some sort of cross-reactivity among T cells). This results in immune activation, and if left unchecked, autoimmune and inflammatory cascades will continue to cause damage throughout the brain and body.

The overall mechanism is the same, but the common theme is that leaky gut leads to the presence of many unwanted materials that make their way into the bloodstream and brain, contributing to autoimmunity, inflammation, blood flow issues, and much more. Theoretically, if your GI system is functioning properly, food allergies shouldn't be an issue, and many individuals are much less sensitive when it comes to certain foods. I've seen individuals who were raised gluten and dairy free from birth; as adults, they have no adverse reactions to these foods. However, most of us suffer from a leaky gut to some degree. It comes down to your specific symptoms, the severity of your symptoms, and whether you're experiencing symptoms that objectively and subjectively correlate to a poor gut. As I said, if you're suffering from any chronic disease, especially Lyme, you shouldn't be eating gluten. Depending on the severity of your symptoms, you should investigate other possible food allergies, like allergies to dairy, soy, and so on. But don't obsess about it.

Simply said, true food allergies contribute to inflammation and immune dysfunction, resulting in damage to numerous bodily systems, organs, and brain regions. I've yet to see an individual come through our doors without one or more of their symptoms linked to immune dysfunction and inflammation. Food allergies are real and further contribute to this immune dysfunction and inflammation.

Most people have a leaky gut to some degree, which usually coincides with malabsorption. But there's a major difference between a nutrient deficiency and body-wide nutrient deficiencies (complete malabsorption). To determine the difference, you must run tests. First, let's look at complete malabsorption of almost every essential amino acid:

	RESULT µM/g creatinine	REFERENCE INTERVAL	PERCENTILE 2.5th 16th 50th 84th 97.5th
Methionine	2.2	7– 35	
Lysine	16	35– 500	
Threonine	27	60– 230	
Leucine	11	18– 70	
Isoleucine	4.2	8– 35	
Valine	13	12– 50	
Phenylalanine	14	25– 75	
Tryptophan	16	20– 75	
Taurine	81	170– 1200	
Cysteine	23	20– 57	
Arginine	7.7	8– 50	
Histidine	190	270– 1150	

You see how nearly every amino acid falls in the bottom 2.5th percentile. I'm not concerned with the values as much as the trend indicating complete malabsorption (body-wide nutrient deficiencies), indicating a leaky gut. The degree of leaky gut is positively correlated with the degree of autoimmunity. The more severe the leaky gut, the more severe the autoimmunity.

Now, that's far different from an actual nutrient deficiency, which is seen below.

	RESULT µM/g creatinine	REFERENCE INTERVAL	PERCENTILE 2.5th 16th 50th 84th 97.5th
Methionine	3.3	7– 35	
Lysine	630	35– 500	
Threonine	120	60– 230	
Leucine	35	18– 70	
Isoleucine	6.8	8– 35	
Valine	31	12– 50	
Phenylalanine	31	25– 75	
Tryptophan	29	20– 75	
Taurine	1390	170– 1200	
Cysteine	11	20– 57	
Arginine	35	8– 50	
Histidine	620	270– 1150	

This is a true nutrient deficiency, in this case, a methionine deficiency, with secondary isoleucine and cysteine deficiencies. Yet the overall absorption is pretty good. This individual probably doesn't have a tremendous issue with leaky gut. This shows how important objective testing can be; more importantly, it shows how important it is to be able to interpret test results and establish a proper treatment plan.

Another growing trend in gut diagnoses is small intestinal bacteria overgrowth (SIBO). This is an issue, but not as much as you may think. Moreover, one of the ways it's treated can actually cause more problems. As explained in the last section, nutrient starvation doesn't work in biofilm treatment, because the biofilm just detaches and finds nutrients elsewhere. The same is often true when you starve the bacterial overgrowth (SIBO) of its food source, sugar, which is one of the conceptual pillars of SIBO treatment nowadays. The overgrowth merely migrates up the GI tract and infects more of your GI system because these overgrowth species want their food; they don't want to die, the same as everything else in the world. In the end, if you have Lyme, a leaky gut, and/or food allergies, you have a high probability of having SIBO. Will treating solely your SIBO get you better? I'd say that's unlikely. Even so, should you starve the body of sugar or vital nutrients such as fiber (a food source for bacteria, both good and bad) to treat SIBO? This is not a revolutionary way of thinking; it is taking a "new" problem and using the same thinking as with every other disorder: starve and kill in hopes of repopulating and healing. Although SIBO is more commonly found in alternative therapies, the approach is still traditional. Solving a new problem with old thinking is not innovating; it is imitating.

OK, let's move on.

When you're sick, your health becomes somewhat of an obsession because you want to get better so badly. Being sick becomes your norm, and it's been years since you've felt like yourself. This leads to you doing more and more research in an attempt to solve your own health riddle. The more research you do, the more you eliminate from your diet. This has this chemical, this has that ingredient, this study shows this, and another shows something else. It can be quite scary. If you have chronic Lyme (or any other chronic disease), you should eliminate gluten completely. I recommend you then eliminate dairy and see whether you notice any additional symptom relief. If so, you should eliminate dairy. Here's where it gets a bit dicey. You could do the same with soy, grains, legumes, nightshades, corn, and more, but there's a balance; you don't want to back yourself into an elimination corner in which you can't go out or over to a friend's house without being stressed about what food will be served. Unless you know from experience or complex testing, it would be a good choice to eliminate gluten and one additional symptom-provoking food.

You cannot live your life in fear. Yes, there are some foods you should just flat-out eliminate, but that's the reality of having a chronic disease like Lyme. Your physician has probably already attached a label to you, "Lyme patient," and you're probably fearful of feeling this way forever. You shouldn't let food become another one of your fears; just make the basic proper choices I've outlined, and let us help you with the rest. At our center, we've seen fear-based diets taken to the extreme. Some individuals avoid everything and limit themselves to drinking food as smoothies or juices, or they take more drastic measures and avoid all lectins completely. We've recently seen more individuals who are avoiding all inflammatory (histamine-provoking) foods. Again, I believe there's a time and a place for everything, and some people may need to eliminate more foods than others because there's no "one size fits all." However, by eliminating more and more foods, you're backing yourself into that elimination corner. Life is about balance, and healing is no different. Most individuals see much improvement in their symptoms by eliminating a few food groups while we correct the other multiple brain and body abnormalities. Diet and nutrition are important steps in healing from Lyme disease. However, you shouldn't let your diet control your life or force you to live in fear. Healing, in large part, is about dropping labels that either you have put on yourself or others have put on you. It's about *not* identifying with the disease. Life is about balance; take it for what it's worth.

Simply said, research into food allergies along with the food we eat can be quite scary. It further contributes to fear and labels placed on you by yourself and/or others, which means it further contributes to your disease state. Don't obsess over food allergies. Dropping fear and labels is one of the most important steps in the healing process.

Many find relief in vegan or vegetarian diets; others prefer a paleo regimen. In the end, your diet depends on your needs, your body, as well as your beliefs.

Hormones and Our Brains

I don't want to delve into hormones too much, because many already know the positive, body-wide effects of many hormones. However, I would like to touch on a few important aspects of hormones that are often overlooked. Here's what I'll talk about in the next section:

- The importance of testing multiple hormones
- Communication between the brain and the hormones
- The importance of hormones in brain function
- The role of MSH, an often-overlooked hormone

First off, as I mentioned when briefly discussing thyroid issues, you can't understand hormones without running an extensive hormonal panel. Let me explain the importance of this concept with a question.

How would you know the difference between a low thyroid and low hormones in general?

Each points to a much different cause; you wouldn't know which cause was more accurate unless you did the testing. If you tested only the thyroid, and it was low or it indicated autoimmunity, could you determine whether this was a localized thyroid issue or a body-wide hormone issue? It would be difficult to come up with a definitive conclusion without more data.

Now, if you tested ten to fifteen different hormones and only the thyroid was low, then it would be easier to draw a more accurate conclusion. If most or all the tested hormones were low, you could also draw a more definitive conclusion, but that conclusion would be much different from the one indicated by one low hormone and ten optimal hormones.

An extensive hormonal panel is necessary because it serves as the basis for understanding the next three functions that are often compromised in Lyme individuals.

I'm going to give you another crash course in communication between the brain and end organs. Have you ever wondered how your ovaries or testicles know when to produce hormones and how much to make? Much is dictated along the communication axis between the sex organs and the brain. The hypothalamus communicates to the pituitary gland (brain region to brain region). Then the pituitary sends signals downstream to hormone-producing organs, such as the thyroid, ovaries, testicles, adrenals, and so on. The end organ then produces the hormone and sends it out to be used. If there's too much or too little of the hormone, communication between the brain and the end organ helps to equalize its production. This system is an intercommunication axis between the brain and its end organs. We find many Lyme individuals have an extremely disrupted axis; this means communication between the brain and the body is often disconnected. The most common disturbance we see among Lyme individuals is a brain that's no longer producing sufficient amounts of hormone signals to the end organs. Often, the result is low body-wide hormone production and use. Not only do we optimize your hormones, but we restore this communication system, as it serves as one of the most fundamental aspects of regulation in your brain and body.

Simply said, testing is the first step and is crucial to understanding hormonal function as well as integrated communication.

Let's move on to the importance of specific hormones and the brain. Many have heard of testosterone but are unaware it plays a major role in the production of dopamine, a pleasure and multifunctional neurotransmitter, in both males and females. Also, testosterone must be paired with other hormones, especially estrogens. Estradiol, the most potent estrogen, is often tested when examining testosterone levels, but estrone (another estrogen) is often overlooked, as are important brain-derived hormones. In males affected by toxicity, testosterone is usually suppressed, with estrone being elevated. Estrone elevation in males indicates poor communication and enzyme activity. (Many times, the estradiol appears normal in this situation.) Below is an example of this phenomenon and the results of just four weeks of treatment.

Before Treatment

Testosterone,Free and Total				
Testosterone, Serum	387		ng/dL	348 - 1197
Estrone, Serum	99	High	pg/mL	12 - 72

After 4 Weeks of Treatment

Testosterone, Serum				
Testosterone, Serum	643		ng/dL	348 - 1197
Estrone, Serum	77	High	pg/mL	12 - 72

You may say, "Yeah, that's what happens when you get old." First, age isn't an excuse to feel terrible and have poor lab values. Second, this individual is in his early twenties. No testosterone or any other hormones were given to him.

Now, in the female brain, estradiol also helps produce dopamine and serotonin while progesterone produces GABA, the number-one calming neurotransmitter. This is part of the reason that when progesterone drops out ten to fifteen years before menopause (in perimenopause), many women develop anxiety and insomnia issues, sometimes resulting in the use of medications like Xanax and Ativan or alcohol. All of these activate the GABA receptor, the same receptor that's activated much less without the production of progesterone. When menopause hits and progesterone, testosterone, and estradiol are basically nonexistent, it's not uncommon for more symptoms to occur, such as pain, fibromyalgia, insomnia, depression, anxiety, night sweats, hot flashes, and many more. Since hormones affect important neurotransmitters, it shouldn't be surprising that upon losing hormones, overall electricity in the brain greatly changes. One of the leading causes of addiction among middle-aged women is hormonal dropout; these individuals are merely self-medicating to calm their overelectrified brains. This is the reason females often increase from one or two glasses of wine to a full bottle or from taking Ativan as needed to eventually requiring it every day. It's not a middle-age crisis; it's usually from hormonal dropout during perimeno-pause and menopause.

Regardless of age or gender, many individuals come to our center with severe neurological symptoms coupled with severe symptoms of electrical imbalance in the brain, causing severe hormone disruption. The most common abnormality is that most, if not all, of their hormones are suppressed. This is another reason addiction is seen in both males and females who aren't even close to their forties or fifties.

Do you see how the symptoms of hormonal suppression and dysregulation are like those of Lyme? Some argue hormones are suppressed in Lyme itself, but how could that happen if they regulate frequently without being directly treated? Hopefully, you realize numerous issues can cause your symptoms—quite accurately, I might add. Yes, the thyroid is important for both the brain and body; yes, DHEA is important for both the brain and body; and I could go on for days. I just want you to understand the concept of how crucial hormones are, not just in the body but in the brain as well.

Simply said, testosterone, estradiol (one of the three estrogens), and progesterone have a dramatic impact on the overall electricity in the brain.

OK, only one more point to cover: melanocyte-stimulating hormone, or MSH. You may have heard of melanin and its relationship to the skin, but MSH is more important in many other aspects of the brain and body. MSH is significantly disrupted by fatty toxins; it's often one of the first hormones disrupted after the initial entry of fatty toxins. When MSH lowers, melatonin lowers (sleep issues increase), sex hormones lower, illnesses become difficult to fight off, GI problems ensue, and adrenal output decreases (17, 101). Not only is it an indication of fatty-toxin toxicity, but it shows how integrated and vital our communication system is and how it must be restored to ensure long-term healing.

Your Genes, Your Imprint: Genetic-Based Therapy

Genetic-based therapy is a growing trend in alternative medicine, especially within the Lyme community. What I mean by genetic-based therapy is therapy that's dictated by your genetics, in which your genetics serves as a basis for your treatment. Individuals come to our clinic with their 23andMe (DNA genetics and testing analysis) results asking about snips, homozygous, and heterozygous (some fancy terms describing genetic profiles), asking us to explain their results. We're always happy to do so, as we truly emphasize and focus on educating individuals because this ensures long-term success. Genetics are just that: education. We never design an entire protocol based solely on your genetics (or your blood type, for that matter). We have some control of the effect of our genetics (by altering gene expression), but for the most part, we can't vastly change our genetics, at least not now. I use genetics as part of the education process because it helps you better understand yourself and your inherent triggers in the world when you go home. It helps you understand what situations exacerbate and provoke your symptoms and what situations will keep you well and improve your quality of life. It also provides some answers as to how you got sick in the first place.

We test for some genetic profiles, including the HLA gene, because it's difficult to keep you well in the long term without knowing whether you possess this gene or not. However, knowing whether you have this gene or not doesn't have any influence on your getting better, regardless of the disadvantages found in your genetics. We get you better whether you have MTHFR issues, the dreaded gene (which is an inaccurate and ridiculous name), or anything else; your genetics merely serve as education for you; after you complete our program, it helps keep you better and helps provide some answers as to why and how you got so sick.

We understand the intricate inner workings of genetics, and we can do extensive tests that we've done in the past. But why do the testing? It won't get you better, and it doesn't serve as the basis for your treatment. We constantly have individuals coming to our clinic saying, "I have this gene or that gene," but it doesn't help get you better. Yes, we test for some genetics, but it wouldn't mean anything if we didn't understand your symptoms and their effects on the brain and body.

All the rage nowadays is the MTHFR gene (methylenetetrahydrofolate reductase, in case you were wondering) and its role in detoxification pathways. Yes, having an issue with this gene can impair your detoxification pathways. But so can an influx of toxins. So can oxidative stress and poor blood flow. So can immune disturbances. And so can imbalances in brain chemistry. All these conditions contribute to impaired methylation, and more importantly, correcting these abnormalities results in vast improvements in methylation pathways. In other words, you'll be fine if you have the MTHFR abnormality and many others, for that matter. I've seen individuals whose previous doctors focused on this gene so much that they became truly fearful of their own genetics. Again, it's another label that needs to be dropped.

The bottom line is that genetics serves merely as an educational tool that helps ensure long-term healing. Testing for numerous types of genetics adds more labels to your disease and only further contributes to your illness. We don't ignore recent discoveries or uses of genetic-based therapies for Lyme patients; however, we don't put all our emphasis on it, either.

Simply said, genetics serves merely as an educational tool that helps ensure long-term healing, but knowing your genetics, in and of itself, will not get you better.

It's All Interconnected: System-to-System Communication

I've discussed this point briefly already, but I'd like to emphasize it once again. Your brain and body are part of an intricate system that fails miserably without communication. The brain communicates among its own regions as well as with other organs and systems. It's crucial to ensure that this communication is functioning properly; otherwise, many problems arise. We see this disrupted communication often in Lyme individuals; however, without testing, it's nearly impossible to discern which systems are out of balance. As I said before, biofilms and their species communicate, and so do your own cells, your own bacteria, and your own systems. It's imperative to restore communication in systems such as the gut-brain axis, the hypothalamic-pituitary-adrenal (HPA) axis, hemispheric brain communication, basal ganglia and cerebellar loops, and numerous others.

I Need More Energy

Every Lyme individual seems to suffer from chronic fatigue. Many have that wired and tired feeling because they're so anxious and aren't getting proper sleep. Even if they're sleeping (which isn't often), the quality of sleep is poor, and they rarely achieve deep sleep. Many focus on the adrenals and boosting energy, but this is a backward approach and doesn't consider a much larger picture. I'll be honest: adrenal fatigue and the adrenals in general are way overblown. It is highly unlikely that your adrenals are the underlying cause of disease and your symptoms. Here is my beef with the adrenals: they're a downstream organ, an end organ. Many signals that dictate much of the activity of the adrenals come from other places. For example, the adrenal rhythm is set by the brain (the hippocampus), and there's system-to-system communication among the adrenals and the hypothalamus and pituitary gland, which are also in the brain. It doesn't make sense to focus on the adrenals and think that could solve the issue; there's more to it. My next beef is that toxicity, other hormones, brain neurotransmitters, inflammation, immune function, and blood flow all have tremendous effects on adrenal output. My final beef for this book is that boosting adrenal activity, energy, and electricity in someone who's already anxious and/or not sleeping isn't a smart idea, as it worsens the symptoms. As I said, it's backward. We restore energy in many individuals without boosting their "get up and go" chemicals and also without boosting their adrenals; we boost energy by restoring electrical activity in their brains and getting them to sleep soundly. Yes, there are herbs that can give you smooth energy, but that doesn't change the fact that you're not sleeping. Sleep is the best way to regulate adrenal activity. Getting someone quality sleep is probably the best tool we have; we believe in correcting the night to heal the day.

Yes, adrenal fatigue is overblown, but energy deficiencies aren't. The adrenals aren't the only way you can boost energy.

After toxins are removed, inflammation is reduced, immune function is normalized, and the brain is balanced electrically, it becomes much easier to boost energy for Lyme individuals. If these things aren't taken care of, much of your efforts to boost energy will be futile. However, sometimes this doesn't alleviate chronic fatigue, which leads to the need for additional tools. We've found that one of the best ways to boost energy and optimize the entire energy system is through mitochondria, glucose, and oxygenation. To be honest, regardless of your energy level, these components should be optimized for the longevity of your brain and body.

Most of the energy we use comes from ATP; it serves as the driving force for much of what we do. ATP is produced in the mitochondria and requires oxygen and glucose (sugar). Most of the time, we see individuals with elevated glucose, yet their diets are pretty good. Upon further examination, we determine they have immune dysfunction, inflammation, and blood-flow issues. Elevated glucose is actually not due to diet but is due to inefficient glucose usage. This also tells us the mitochondria are suboptimal as well and in need of some help. Along with addressing the immune system, reducing inflammation, and promoting better blood flow, we directly help the mitochondria with basic tools such as CoQ10, PQQ, and high-quality fatty acids. We also have our own specific tools as well. In the end, it's crucial to optimize glucose utilization and help boost mitochondrial activity to enhance ATP production, energy, and overall brain and body function.

Simply said, the best way to focus on energy and chronic fatigue is through the mitochondria, oxygen delivery, and glucose utilization and not the adrenals.

What about Infections? What about Lyme Disease?

All right! Lyme disease—that's what the whole book's about. In all fairness, I should talk about the possibility of Lyme playing a major role in your symptoms because it's possible, although implausible, as it happens only less than 10 percent of the time. Many people assume I don't know how to kill Lyme, and that's the reason I don't go after it. This couldn't be further from the truth. I know so much about Lyme, about biofilms, and about die-off that they're the reasons I know you shouldn't kill it. By now, you should agree. If not, don't worry; you still have a few chapters left to come around. In all transparency, I do know our world is not black and white, and there's a possibility that infections could be a major cause of your symptoms. I saved less than 10 percent of this section to discuss Lyme itself because you only should kill Lyme less than 10 percent of the time—seems fitting, doesn't it? In the past year, it's been less than 5 percent, but that's OK; I'll use the 10 percent figure anyway.

After you adequately address blood flow, the brain, inflammation, hormones, the GI system, mental-emotional disturbances, the immune system, autoimmunity, toxicity, and a whole bunch of other stuff I've discussed in this section, and your symptoms still aren't resolved, then you may have a case for Lyme playing a major role in your symptoms. So many individuals feel that a Lyme diagnosis is everything, as though Lyme were the answer to all their problems, but it's not. I hope I've provided enough information so you can take a step back and honestly look at your own symptoms. I hope I've provided enough information so you understand that many other issues I've discussed can explain your symptoms much better than Lyme itself. The reason we get you better without killing Lyme 90 percent of the time is that Lyme isn't the cause of your symptoms 90 percent of the time. People seek and desire one cause to explain everything, but that's not reality for any chronic disease. If you look at multiple different possibilities, multiple different causalities, you begin to realize the symptoms you've associated with Lyme aren't Lyme at all; they're the result of these other causalities. How do you truly know that Lyme is causing all your symptoms, especially when testing reveals other abnormalities? Testing allows for our approach, and individuals getting better time and time again proves that testing is essential to long-term health. Once you understand this, we devise a plan that gets you better quickly and safely.

To finish off my examples before getting to the case studies at the end of the book, here's an instance in which immune function was optimized so well that this individual's **Lyme marker went negative after just four weeks** of treatment. (And yes, we did a whole lot of other modalities besides boosting immune function to accomplish this.)

Before Treatment

TESTS	RESULT	FLAG	UNITS	REFERENCE INTERVAL
CD4/CD8 Ratio Profile				
Absolute CD 4 Helper	539		/uL	359 - 1519
% CD 4 Pos. Lymph.	49.0		%	30.8 - 58.5
Abs. CD 8 Suppressor	221		/uL	109 - 897
% CD 8 Pos. Lymph.	20.1		%	12.0 - 35.5
CD4/CD8 Ratio	2.44			0.92 - 3.72
WBC	4.9		x10E3/uL	3.4 - 10.8
Abs.CD8-CD57+ Lymphs	30	Low	/uL	60 - 360

After 4 Weeks of Treatment

TESTS	RESULT	FLAG	UNITS	REFERENCE INTERVAL
CD4/CD8 Ratio Profile				
Absolute CD 4 Helper	728		/uL	359 - 1519
% CD 4 Pos. Lymph.	42.8		%	30.8 - 58.5
Abs. CD 8 Suppressor	316		/uL	109 - 897
% CD 8 Pos. Lymph.	18.6		%	12.0 - 35.5
CD4/CD8 Ratio	2.30			0.92 - 3.72
WBC	6.9		x10E3/uL	3.4 - 10.8
Abs.CD8-CD57+ Lymphs	71		/uL	60 - 360

Yes, I understand a CD57 isn't 100 percent accurate in diagnosing Lyme, but it's a good indication of the chronic nature of your Lyme as well as your chronic infectious load in general. Moreover, when you pair this immune value with the other two values seen above, you become more confident in concluding immune function has greatly improved across the board. You see how it went from being positive at 30 cells/uL to negative at 71 cells/uL. Moreover, this individual's CD4:CD8 ratio improved (got closer to 2.0), and his overall immune function greatly improved, with CD4 cells/uL increasing from 539 to 728 and CD8 cells/uL increasing from 221 to 316. This individual's immune function was nearly completely restored in less than a month of treatment.

But hey, I'll give you some information (albeit briefly because it's not really necessary) on that 10 (or 5) percent, as I promised.

Lyme is a bear to treat, as you've probably already realized. To properly address Lyme, it takes many months, and you shouldn't administer too many killing days within a given period. Whether it's vitamin C, hydrogen peroxide, herbs, essential oils, liposomal vitamins and herbal blends, enzymes, or whatever else, they all elicit kills by breaching biofilms. Thus, between these days, you should be resting and detoxing from opening the biofilm. Many of you already know this, but I hope you now understand the additional measures that must be addressed to account for everything existing within biofilms. I've heard too many stories about individuals with regimented schedules determining when and how to take supplements, herbs, oils, and foods down to the half hour and accounting for the entire day; this is no way to live. Even if you get better, I guarantee you will live in fear of Lyme forever and probably relapse multiple times. You will unnecessarily battle Lyme for the rest of your life. Again, this is no way to live; don't let yourself become a victim of any disease.

Any type of Lyme treatment should be undertaken only with a strong, mentally sound individual because of the length and tedious nature of the ensuing treatment. Also, Lyme is rarely the only infection you have. What I mean is there are many coinfections commonly associated with Lyme, yet these coinfections don't function in the same fashion as Lyme, even though many build biofilms like Lyme. Additional measures must be taken to account for the differences between infections, in addition to everything else that's within biofilms. For example, infections that tend to be located within your cells (intercellular pathogens) should be addressed differently than infections located just outside your cells (extracellular pathogens), and both infections should be handled differently than a Lyme infection. Some parasites function differently than bacteria, and viruses differ from both bacteria and parasites in many ways. Also, you must attack one type of pathogen at a time. Assembling a plan that attempts to wipe out all pathogens at one time is scientifically implausible, dangerous, and dumb.

My last point is illustrated by a short story. When I was in college, hornets built a nest just outside my front door. I had to walk past them, in and out of my house, every day. I told those hornets, "If you sting me, I'm taking down your nest. If you don't sting me, I won't take it down." Yeah, I know that's a bit weird that I said that statement out loud at the time, but that's how I felt about the hornets, and that's how I feel about Lyme disease. If it isn't stinging you, if it isn't attacking you, why go after it? Especially when there are so many other issues that need fixing, and they're a lot easier and less harmful to treat. To continue that point, if the hornets were to sting you, if the Lyme were to attack and pose a viable threat, then you would take down the nest. But you would take down only one nest. You wouldn't go on a hunt around the exterior of your house, wiping out all the hornet nests you could find. What I am trying to say is if you're provoked, then go after your Lyme, but go after some of the Lyme. You don't (and actually can't) go after all the Lyme. When you do attack Lyme, you must break open the biofilm, which means you'll need expertise on biofilms and all the havoc inside them.

Additionally, when I am speaking about infections and pathogenic exposure, I mean pathogens hiding within biofilms. Any free-floating parasites, harmful bacteria, or damaging viruses contributing to your symptoms are eliminated with our therapy. However, it's done without opening the biofilm and, more importantly, without causing die-off.

The bottom line remains that this treatment isn't likely, and you won't need to plan for months, even years, of therapy at our center, because Lyme isn't the cause of your symptoms more than 90 percent of the time.

Simply said, you don't have to kill Lyme more than 90 percent of the time, but after you exhaust and adequately address every option in this section, Lyme *may* be an issue. Regardless, killing Lyme is a tedious endeavor that has a significant effect mentally, emotionally, and physically on any individual.

How Are These Factors Used and Addressed?

Each issue discussed in each chapter plays a significant role in your Lyme treatment. Each must be understood and examined, both qualitatively and quantitatively. Now it's time to use the tools and address any abnormalities of concern. Each tool has a different value to each person, and the tools must be used in a specific order. There's a method- a scientific, systemized method - because tools don't do much of anything if you don't know how to use them.

How do we calm the brain? How do we remove toxins? How do we enhance blood flow? How do we utilize this information, all the data that's been gathered? How do we develop a unique plan for you?

In the next few chapters, I'll discuss our methods and how each of them is designed to address everything that I've discussed throughout this section. You may think you've tried something that incorporated some of these methods, or maybe you've tried something similar, but you haven't. Our 100 percent all-natural method and system is patent pending, so I know you've never tried anything like this.

IV Therapy

The most efficient and potent way to deliver nutrients to the body is, arguably, intravenously (through an IV), or directly into the blood stream. IV therapy has a few unique qualities that separate it from many other nutrient-delivery techniques:

- It tends to be more potent; thus it tends to have the biggest effect.
- The dose is much more controlled.
- It bypasses the gut and GI system.
- It works quickly and saves time.

Since the nutrient goes directly into the bloodstream, you don't rely on the GI system to break down and absorb nutrients; that step is bypassed. Most individuals suffering from Lyme have poor GI systems and a compromised ability to break down and absorb vital nutrients. Often, supplementation alone isn't potent enough to heal your symptoms. We also control the exact dose you receive as well as the potency and duration of the nutrients delivered. Utilizing our 100 percent all-natural IV therapy is one reason our treatment time is so much quicker. (The main reason is we don't treat Lyme to get you better.)

Many people tell me, "I've tried IV therapy, and it didn't work. What makes yours so different?"

My best answer to that is "Everything." I honestly don't mean to be arrogant, but you haven't tried anything like our therapy, including our IVs. It's 100 percent all-natural and patent pending.

Here's what separates our IV therapy from others you've tried. Our IV therapy accomplishes the following:

- Calms the brain down, restores brain electricity and neurotransmitter systems
- Calms vagus nerve activity, helps calm the immune system
- Provides metabolic support for your brain and cells
- Restores receptivity
- Replenishes nutrition
- Removes environmental/industrial toxins

We get you better, all naturally, without the use of drugs, without killing your Lyme, and in far less time. You must be ready for treatment and trust our process. You may think it's impossible to accomplish those goals, especially in a matter of weeks, but it's not. This is our specialty, our passion; we get you better because we know the mechanisms and we understand the data and the science, which gives us the ability to get you better. I'll show results of real individuals at the end of this section.

Simply said, our IV therapy focuses on replenishing your brain and body, removing toxins, and restoring your brain's electrical activity. It's totally different from any experience you've ever had.

Is My IV Therapy Unique to Me?

Another common question we get is "Is my IV therapy unique to me?

Yes.

We specifically design every IV for each individual based on his or her testing results, questionnaires, and symptoms; our physical/neurological exam; and our experience. Each IV is unique to the individual, and sometimes it changes weekly or even daily.

Oral Supplementation

With Lyme disease, you seem to constantly be fighting an uphill battle. IV therapy alone often doesn't provide enough relief, and it's difficult to start winning the battle against Lyme without oral supplements. We like to hammer home the same concepts when you're not at our center as well; thus, we use supplements to further enhance these concepts emphasized in our IV therapy. As many Lyme individuals have compromised GI systems, the overuse of supplementation isn't useful. We try to limit our supplementation in both the short term and long term because our goal is to get the maximum healing effects in the least amount of time. Moreover, taking supplements and/or prescription medications every day just further masks what's going on. We heal your true symptoms by minimizing your supplements and by detoxing you off your prescription drugs. Supplementation is an important part of our therapy because it allows us to tackle additional issues, especially blood flow, inflammation, and immunity. However, we use different kinds and quantities of supplements throughout the healing process, with the end goal of lowering your supplement use toward the end of your healing process. In the long term, the goal is and always will be to get you better.

Getting Back to the Basics

My overall goal is the least amount of supplementation possible, hopefully zero medications, while still achieving your healing goals. This isn't an unreachable goal; we accomplish it with the overwhelming majority of our Lyme individuals. Long-term success is deeply rooted in education as well; however, in the end, getting back to basics is what keeps you better. Once we remove your toxic burden, regulate your immune system, optimize your hormones and boost your blood flow; you'll get better and stay better. Once we heal your brain and body and lift the burden of disease from your shoulders, you finally return to your life and to doing the things you want to do. I assure you that you'll be able to maintain these achievements on your own, with the basics you've learned from this book.

Some chapters are short, but I felt obligated to mention the topics in them. I also know you're aware of the importance of these issues, but when you're sick, you lose the little things: you stop going outside, you stop exercising, you stop everything. I remember when I first started feeling well, the only things I wanted to do were the basics: I wanted to enjoy a meal, to sit in the sun, to take a walk, to listen to the birds, and to exercise. We restore your connection to these activities, to the basics, to nature, because it ensures long-term healing and a lifestyle change both physically and mentally. Don't correlate the length of these sections with their importance. The following are some of the easiest, the most often overlooked, and the most necessary steps for your healing process.

WE MUST GET YOU TO MOVE

I could tell you obvious benefits such as blood flow, brain help, immunity, genetic expression, cardiovascular health, and beyond, but the bottom line is you must exercise. Find what works best for your body, your brain, and your lifestyle, but you must exercise; it's crucial in the healing process for Lyme and any other chronic disease.

A little while back, I was researching complex biochemical reasons for the poor oxygenation and blood-flow values in individuals at our clinic, when I realized I was ignoring the obvious. These individuals used to be active, and now they were nearly completely stagnant in all aspects, both mentally and physically. Exercise is by far the best tool for boosting blood flow.

Many may not be able to exercise in the traditional sense, often from complications of Lyme, but we'll give you a plan that meets your needs and your abilities. Whether it's myofascial release, resistance-band therapy, light cardio, or full-on, high-intensity interval training, wherever you're at, we'll meet you there and then push you a bit beyond. We've determined the proper intensity as well as the proper time at which exercise should be introduced because as with everything, if exercise is done improperly, symptoms will worsen. Even exercise requires more than just simple understanding.

Nature and the Sun

Getting back to the environment and back to nature is probably the easiest and one of the best healing tools. Get outside; go for a walk, a hike, or a run. Get in the sun, soak up the energy, and get some warmth to your bones. Get in the water; a lake or the ocean. Go for a swim, or just float there; I don't care. But you must do it. Getting back to nature gets you better all by itself.

Hydrotherapy

Hydrotherapy is a classic technique in natural medicine, but it's often equated with just colon hydrotherapy or colonics. Colonics is often necessary if you're going through Lyme kills, as massive amounts of toxins will dry your bowels and tend to cause constipation. Because you must rid your body of excess toxins, many clinics want to ensure the elimination by using colonics. Colonics aren't necessary if you don't administer Lyme-kill therapy. Hydrotherapy is much more than colonics, and these classic techniques have been used for centuries and prove to be helpful for Lyme individuals.

We design a hydrotherapy protocol that meets your needs, and much of the time, it's as simple as a basic contrast protocol. When you have heat, you draw circulation, or blood flow, to the area. When you have cold, you push circulation away from the area. If you alternate between hot and cold (hence contrast), you create a mechanical pump in the area. This works wonders for circulation and temperature sensitivity, so don't overlook the benefits of hydrotherapy. Postural orthostatic tachycardia syndrome (POTS), an autonomic disorder, is common among chronic Lyme individuals. We've found you can exercise the brain (the hypothalamus), which is responsible for a lot of autonomic functions, by using contrast hydrotherapy. When contrast hydrotherapy is used in conjunction with other tools outlined in this section (especially fatty-toxin toxicity), POTS often proves to be a disorder of communication, not a permanent condition. Through our hydrotherapy protocols, many report feeling more refreshed, having less fatigue, and having less sensitivity to temperature. Hydrotherapy is a low-cost, low-time healing tool with not much risk, so of course we use it.

So Many Other Tools

We blend multiple ways of thinking, which include multiple ways of viewing medicine. (And yes, that includes allopathic/Western medicine.) We use a variety of ayurvedic and Chinese herbs, but usually not extensively, as they are often used to boost immune function; since we accomplish this naturally with our protocol, we tend not to need immune-boosting Eastern herbs. We see homeopathy, acupuncture, and craniosacral therapy as great tools for shifting energy, releasing energy, and providing relief from symptoms, especially in the mental-emotional realm—quite effectively, I might add. Chiropractic work is an important tool in boosting blood flow to the brain as well as correcting structural deficiencies contributing greatly to tension/structural headaches, migraines, and chronic pain. We are closely associated with many experienced practitioners who use these techniques every day. So whether it's tinctures, herbs, teas, or electromagnetic or frequency therapy, whatever it is, if it's indicated, we'll use it. If it helps you, we'll use it.

Let me end this section with a recap of what must be analyzed and done appropriately in Lyme individuals:

- Addressing mind-body connection
- Balancing neurotransmitters and electricity in the brain

- Addressing underactive and overactive brain regions
- Restoring receptivity
- Enhancing mitochondrial efficiency
- Regulating immunity/stopping autoimmune reactions
- Diagnosing and educating individuals on genetic abnormalities
- Removing environmental/industrial toxins
- Reducing inflammation
- Optimizing hormonal function
- Increasing circulation (blood flow)
- Replenishing nutrition and correcting nutritional deficiencies
- Removing food allergens from diet
- Educating individuals on lifestyle, diet, and exercise
- Replenishing the gut lining and beneficial gut bacteria
- Restoring system-to-system communication

That's all step one.

When we work together to fix these issues, you get better. It's inevitable, but we must work together, and you must be truly ready to get better. This program isn't something for which you just show up and get an IV and take supplements. There is a lot of work involved from both of us. Every individual who's gotten better has worked tremendously hard to do so. We also match that hard work, determination, and discipline, which ensures you get and stay better. As I said, this is step one.

Many centers try to establish a generic formula for treating individuals, but nearly all issues must be addressed simultaneously in a specific fashion to heal Lyme individuals. Some issues play a larger role than others in Lyme individuals, but a concurrent, holistic approach is vital. I hope you've noticed that none of our steps involve killing Lyme; it's not necessary to get you better.

Now let's see how all this comes together in real individuals.

Real People, Real Results

The following case studies are true stories of real individuals treated at our center. They are real cases of people who told us what their symptoms were upon arrival. I show the improvement of each individual using his or her own assessments and our concrete, objective treatments, including eliminating medications and reducing supplements. I'll mention some of their tests as I discuss their stories, but in the end, the test results don't matter. These people feel better, and that's all that will ever matter.

Many clinics show only their superstar patients and never show their norms. Clinics show videos of wheelchair miracles, however a few months after treatment, some return to their original debilitating condition – sometimes even worse. I could have chosen to do the same, but that's not reality. I selected these people on purpose to represent the greater population of the individuals that we treat. Yes, there are plenty more individuals; these are the types of people we see every day. Again, they allow you to conceptually understand Lyme disease and not just what's possible but what's probable. These are real people from all over the world, with various backgrounds, with different ages and different genders, with a multitude of unique and general symptoms. Not every person experiences a 100 percent recovery, mainly because healing the chronically sick takes time. However, each of these people attained his or her goal of symptom reduction and an improvement in his or her quality of life. I'd love to tell you everyone dramatically recovers in a matter of days, but that's not the norm either. Some do, but most do not. Some improve between 90 and 100 percent, and some improve between 50 and 60 percent; some improve quickly, and some take a bit more time; but the large majority of our individuals feel they improved between 60 and 80 percent after completing just four to six weeks of our treatment protocol; this is our initial program length. I will limit the background stories for individuals because I want you to pay attention to their viewpoints on their own symptoms as well as noticing their supplementation and medication reductions. What I say is not as relevant, because it's an individual's perspective that matters and allows for true long-term healing.

As I've stated, I could have selected all our superstar individuals, individuals who recovered between 90 and 100 percent, but I chose cases to represent the majority, which is most realistic. Each person selected was chosen to highlight something specific because, as always, I want you to learn. For example, you'll notice most individuals discussed are women; that is because between 70 and 80 percent of the individuals we see for Lyme are women. This isn't to say men don't have Lyme; that would be a ridiculous statement. I'm just giving you our information. Another point is that most individuals were unable to work due to the debilitating nature of their symptoms; in our clinic, this is true for about 60 percent of individuals. More than half of the individuals discussed were on multiple medications, which is also representative of the individuals at our center. Most of individuals listed below are from different demographics and geographical locations, because I hope by now you realize Lyme can affect pretty much anyone, anywhere. The treatment time for each person is also listed below; however, any individual who was treated for more than four to six weeks was detoxing from pharmaceutical medications. These individuals returned for additional treatment after they went home for a month or so, which is a necessary part of our therapy. Going home and resting between therapies verifies that their treatment successes are real and sustainable because of their tremendous hard work and compliance with our program's protocol while at our center and, more importantly, after they return home. Every individual put in the hard work necessary to get better. The healing process isn't just "Come in and get an IV, take some supplements, and go home." The healing process requires work; it's a team effort. I'll also discuss what our testing and analyses revealed from a physiological perspective, so you understand why it's impossible to develop a cookie-cutter program—everyone's symptoms and tests are vastly different. Yet what we have developed is the knowledge and understanding for each tool I've discussed in this section. I'll tell you the primary, secondary, and tertiary issues in each of these individuals from our perspective for you to get an idea of our process. In the end, we give you tools and put them in the proper place to give you the best chance to succeed, but your body dictates its usage of these tools, and you and your body do the healing. We help everyone make that leap, if he or she is ready, just as all the individuals below have done.

LYME DISEASE: THE TRUE REALITY

The first individual is a female from California in her midfifties. She had suffered from anxiety for upward of twenty years, although recently it had become much worse. She rarely had restful sleep, and she experienced severe pain in her wrists, hips, and more. She received past diagnoses ranging from Lyme disease to fibromyalgia. Below, you see what her symptoms were when she arrived; after six weeks of treatment, this individual saw great improvement in three of her top four symptoms.

Before Treatment

- Symptoms
  - Insomnia/Sleep Issues – 9
  - Anxiety – 9
  - Pain – 9
  - GI Issues – 7

- Medications
  - None

After 6 Weeks of Treatment

- Symptoms
  - Insomnia/Sleep Issues – 2
  - Anxiety – 2
  - Pain – 3-4
  - GI Issues – 6-7

- Medications
  - None

Through questionnaires and quantitative testing, we concluded the following:

- Primary abnormalities
  - Neurotransmitter imbalance
  - Hormonal imbalance
  - Inflammation
- Secondary abnormalities
  - Leaky gut syndrome—food allergies previously addressed
  - Blood flow

After her brain and hormonal system started to become balanced, her sleep dramatically improved. The anxiety and pain reduced but not to the levels they are today. We continued to work on inflammation and detoxification (although her fatty-toxin load wasn't high) while further optimizing her brain chemistry. After six weeks of treatment, her symptoms dropped to what is seen above. We simultaneously worked on her neurotransmitters, hormones, inflammation, and blood-flow issues while putting her GI symptoms on the back burner. Since her GI symptoms weren't resolved by our working on all the issues, we set her up with a long-term GI program and subsequently stayed in contact with her, as well as referring her to a physician in her area.

This next individual is a female in her early twenties from Florida who suffered from anxiety and sleep issues for about eight years before taking a turn for the worse about four years prior to her arrival at our center. She had previously sought treatment for Lyme, and she underwent more than seven months of seemingly endless unnecessary kill treatments while spending tens of thousands of dollars. She ended up on multiple medications but was still suffering from severe insomnia, anxiety, brain fog, and head pressure. After thirteen weeks of treatment, most, if not all, of her symptoms improved.

Before Treatment	After 13 Weeks of Treatment
• Symptoms – Rated as 1-10, with 10 being unbearable	• Symptoms
o Brain Fatigue – 7-8	o Brain Fatigue – 3
o Body Fatigue – 7-8	o Body Fatigue – 4
o Head Pressure – 9	o Head Pressure – 2
o Insomnia/Sleep Issues – 9	o Insomnia/Sleep Issues – 3
o Brain Fog/Memory – 8	o Brain Fog/Recalling Information – 2
• Medications	• Medications
o Lyrica – 300mg Daily	o None
o Rilutek – 100mg Daily	
o Temazepam	
o Clonazepam	
• Supplements	• Supplements
o 90 capsules total	o 30 capsules total per day

As you can see, she's no longer on any medications, and her supplement total has dropped to one-third of her original amount. Sometimes when individuals come off medications, symptoms take much longer to improve because the brain and body are learning to adapt to their new environment, an environment without drugs. In this case, all her symptoms improved, but it took more than twice as long as it did for the previous individual, mainly because we needed to detox her from the pharmaceuticals to ensure long-term healing.

From our perspective, we concluded the following:

- Primary abnormalities
  - Pharmaceuticals
  - Mind-body
  - Blood flow
  - Neurotransmitter imbalance

In our opinion, although there were no secondary or tertiary abnormalities, it took much longer to correct the brain and blood-flow issues because of the inherent hurdle of her being on multiple prescription medications. Since these issues began in her teens and she was currently not working, it was imperative to work with her on reestablishing the mind-body connection.

The next individual I'd like to discuss is in her early twenties as well. She's from Ohio and has suffered chronic migraines for seven years. Because of this excruciating pain, she ended up taking opiate pain medications for years. Eventually she was diagnosed with Lyme disease and has spent upward of $500,000.00 on failed treatments. Before her arrival, sleep was nonexistent, even with her medications. She was also experiencing total body seizures a few times a week when she arrived at our clinic, walking with a cane. After six weeks of treatment, she was medication-free, her seizures had subsided, and her mobility had greatly improved. However, her pain had not really diminished much, and sleep was still an issue. In this case, we expect her to make a full recovery, but her brain hasn't caught up to her body; it's still relearning how to live without medications. I threw in this case at the last minute as I was finishing up this book to show that sometimes it takes more time for symptoms to improve. Sometimes it takes more time for the brain to heal and relearn how to tackle life once again. She has many of the tools she needs, and we've given her a long-term program to follow, but we feel she doesn't need any more in-clinic treatment. I expect when we check in with her in the future, she'll continue to experience symptom improvement, but

I'll probably have an update for you after this book is published, so check with me then. Here are her symptoms, medications, and supplements before and after treatment.

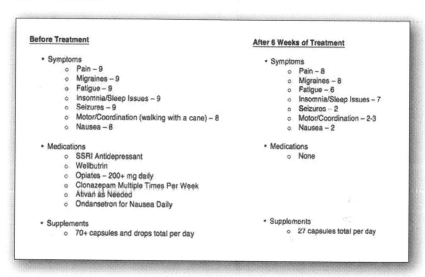

Before Treatment

- Symptoms
    - Pain – 9
    - Migraines – 9
    - Fatigue – 9
    - Insomnia/Sleep Issues – 9
    - Seizures – 9
    - Motor/Coordination (walking with a cane) – 8
    - Nausea – 8

- Medications
    - SSRI Antidepressant
    - Wellbutrin
    - Opiates – 200+ mg daily
    - Clonazepam Multiple Times Per Week
    - Ativan as Needed
    - Ondansetron for Nausea Daily

- Supplements
    - 70+ capsules and drops total per day

After 6 Weeks of Treatment

- Symptoms
    - Pain – 8
    - Migraines – 8
    - Fatigue – 6
    - Insomnia/Sleep Issues – 7
    - Seizures – 2
    - Motor/Coordination – 2-3
    - Nausea – 2

- Medications
    - None

- Supplements
    - 27 capsules total per day

Our analyses showed the following:

- Primary abnormalities
    - Pharmaceuticals
    - Mind-body
    - Toxicity
    - Blood flow
    - Neurotransmitter imbalance
- Secondary abnormalities
    - Malabsorption, candida overgrowth
    - Hormonal imbalance

This next individual is also female, and she's in her mid-thirties and lives in Maryland. Pain, sleep, and fatigue were her main symptoms, and she had previously received a diagnosis for Lyme and had spent more than $100,000.00 on her previous Lyme treatment alone. You can see her improvement below.

Before Treatment	After 13 Weeks of Treatment
• Symptoms	• Symptoms
○ Brain Fog/Memory – 8-9	○ Brain Fog/Memory – 1
○ Pain – 9-10	○ Pain – 5
○ Insomnia/Sleep Issues – 8-9	○ Insomnia/Sleep Issues – 3
○ Fatigue – 8-10	○ Fatigue – 4
○ GI Issues – 7	○ GI Issues – 5
○ Depression – 8-10	○ Depression - 1
• Medications	• Medications
○ Clonazepam Daily	○ Marinol once per day
○ Marinol up to 5 times per day	
○ Vyvanse	
○ Ondansetron for Nausea	
○ Hydrocortisone	
○ Rilutek (ALS Medication)	
• Supplements	• Supplements
○ 109 capsules total per day	○ 45 capsules total per day

This is a case in which the individual's brain and body began to reteach themselves after months of hard work - on her part - in between and following her treatment at our center. She still suffers from pain, although it's reduced. Now that she sleeps better, she has more energy, and her depression has lifted, the pain is also much easier to deal with. She's now progressing steadily and getting back into work again.

Our perspective was as follows:

- Primary abnormalities
  - Pharmaceuticals
  - Mind-body
  - Inflammation
  - Blood flow
  - Neurotransmitter imbalance
  - Hormonal imbalance
- Secondary abnormalities
  - Malabsorption, GI inflammation

I checked with this patient prior to publication, and she is now working consistently, and is no longer taking Marinol. As I've stated, we value testing because it allows us to understand each individual, and it always helps to quantitate improvement from an objective perspective. We'd love to see everyone improve both from his or her own perspective and from a laboratory perspective; however, that's not always the case. This next individual's labs didn't improve for the most part, yet her symptoms did. She is in her mid-twenties and resides in New York. We continued to check on her months after her treatment, and she's continued to improve. Although if we conducted testing today, I'd expect improvement from her original values, at the time this wasn't the case. Her values seemed to indicate Lyme, although you can never be sure, but she'd never been diagnosed or received treatment for Lyme. She did, however, suffer from the very symptoms Lyme individuals endure. These symptoms included insomnia, depression, anxiety, and migraines. There's no difference between this individual and many of the other people we see, except for those with an actual diagnosis. However, she was in a much better position mentally because she hadn't spent years receiving treatment for Lyme, which probably would have made her symptoms worse, and more importantly, she hadn't spent years with a label of Lyme. You can see that largely because of these factors, her treatment time was only three weeks.

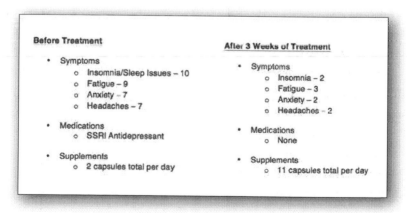

As mentioned, her lab results got worse after she completed treatment, yet her symptoms greatly improved, and she's working full time. Again, it's about how you feel, not always what the numbers say.

This last person I'll show you was one of the first individuals who ever came to our center. We have an additional aftercare program, and we still like to stay updated on all our individuals as best we can. He's from Ohio and had spent well over half a million dollars on previous treatments. As with many of our individuals, he endured the hardships of Lyme treatment, telling us that his daughter would help him walk to the bathroom just so he could vomit. He had suffered for more than ten years before arriving at our center.

Before Treatment	After 4 Weeks of Treatment
• Symptoms	• Symptoms
○ Muscle Aches – 9	○ Muscle Aches – 3
○ Inability to Exercise – 9	○ Inability to Exercise – 3
○ Insomnia/Sleep Issues – 8	○ Insomnia/Sleep Issues – 1
○ Anxiety – 7	○ Anxiety – 2
○ Fatigue – 8	○ Fatigue – 2
○ Brain Fog – 7	○ Brain Fog/Memory - 3
• Medications	• Medications
○ Blood Pressure Medications	○ Blood Pressure Medications
○ Ativan 3x/week	

The symptoms Lyme individuals experience are something you wouldn't wish on anyone; I truly hope you realize I'm not diminishing your symptoms by any means. I'm trying to show you there's a much better, more accurate explanation for them. I'm trying to show you there's a better way, a method that requires far less time without the debilitating symptoms of die-off. I hope this book reaches everyone who's suffering not just from Lyme but from any chronic disease. This information must not fall on deaf ears. It needs to be heard, and it needs to be understood. At a minimum, you should understand there's another option; I never want anyone to feel that no one can help you. We can help you get well. If you're willing to work with us, there's no telling how far you will reach. I can't stand to watch people suffer, especially knowing how much we can help. I want you to take hold of your life once again, and we'll do everything possible to ensure that happens.

What about Other Chronic Diseases and Disorders?

Although this entire book is about Lyme, it speaks to much more than Lyme disease. Although I'm biased because I wrote the book, there's no doubt that the method and procedure we use to heal Lyme is the same method employed for all our individuals suffering from chronic diseases. Our protocol is designed for a multitude of neurological and autoimmune conditions, ranging from drug detox to chronic migraines, even to multiple sclerosis and severe memory and mobility impairment; it just so happens many Lyme individuals are drawn or referred to our center. Everything I've outlined in this book applies to nearly all chronic diseases and autoimmune conditions. All chronic diseases have autoimmunity, inflammation, toxicity, brain imbalances, and so forth. This isn't the method to treat just Lyme; this is the method to treat all chronic diseases. Every chronic disease requires a multifaceted approach from all possible angles. Sure, other treatments are successful; I'm not questioning that, by any means. A multifaceted approach is the only way to ensure the best possible outcome for long-term healing. This process gets people better, no matter the condition. Every condition we treat goes through the same process; all conditions require testing, all individuals are seen every day, and all conditions are addressed using every tool I've outlined in this section. The tools themselves don't change from person to person. The biggest difference seen from individual to individual is our ability to understand the order in which issues are addressed and to know which issues are playing the most significant roles.

Medicine is in a position to change, and current science undoubtedly allows this to occur; it allows for a better way. The days of treating Lyme disease and other chronic ailments with antibiotics and prescription medications are over. We provide you with the answers and results you've been desperately seeking for years. Medicine is failing many of you, and you know in your heart that there's a better way, a different way; we're here to meet that need, to provide a way out. We'll transform our world by transforming the individual, one at a time, by helping everyone, not just someone. With all who are suffering, one person is not nearly enough.

Works Cited

1. Sternbach G., and Dibble C. "Willy Burgdorfer: Lyme Disease." *Journal of Emergency Medicine* 14.5 (1996): 63–4.

2. Scrimenti R., and Scrimenti M. "Lyme Disease Redux: The Legacy of Sven Hellerstrom." *Journal of Spirochetal and Tick-borne Diseases* 8. Fall/Winter (2001). Reprinted from *Wisconsin Medical Journal* 92.1 (1993): 20–1.

3. Wu B. "Johns Hopkins Launches First Ever Center to Focus on Lyme Disease." *The Science Times*, May 27, 2015 http://www.sciencetimes.com/articles/6/25/20150527/johns-hopkins-launches-first-ever-center-to-focus-on-lyme-disease.htm.

4. Centers for Disease Control and Prevention. "Publication of Summary of Notifiable Diseases—United States, 2013." *Morbidity and Mortality Weekly Report* 60.53 July 5, 2013: 1099–100. http://www.cdc.gov/mmwr/pdf/wk/mm6053.pdf.

5. Centers for Disease Control and Prevention. "CDC Provides Estimate of Americans Diagnosed with Lyme Disease Each Year." Press Release August 19, 2013. http://www.cdc.gov/media/releases/2013/p0819-lyme-disease.html.

6. Joo H-S., and Otto M. "Molecular Basis of In-vivo Biofilm Formation by Bacterial Pathogens." *Chemistry & Biology* 19.12 (2012): 1503–13.

7. MacDonald A. *Biofilms of Borrelia Burfdorferi and Clinical Applications for Chronic Borreliosis.* PowerPoint presentation, May 17, 2008. Lyme Disease Symposium, University of New Haven, New Haven, Connecticut.

8.   Stricker R., and Johnson L. "Lyme Disease: The Next Decade." *Infection and Drug Resistance* 4 (2011): 1–9.

9.   Centers for Disease Control and Prevention. "Transmission." March 4, 2015. http://www.cdc.gov/lyme/transmission/.

10.   Stonehouse A., Studdiford J., and Henry C. "An Update on the Diagnosis and Treatment of Early Lyme Disease: Focusing on the Bull's Eye, You May Miss the Mark." *The Journal of Emergency Medicine* 39.5 (2010): 147–51.

11.   Schaible U., Gay S., Museteanu C., Kramer M., Zimmer G., Eichmann K., Museteanu U., and Simon M. "Lyme Borreliosis in the Severe Combined Immunodeficiency (scid) Mouse Manifests Predominantly in the Joints, Heart, and Liver." *The American Journal of Pathology.* 137.4 (1990): 811–20.

12.   Garcia-Monco J., Frey H., Villar B., Golightly M, and Benach J. "Lyme Disease Concurrent with Human Immunodeficiency Virus Infection." *The American Journal of Medicine* 87.3 (1989): 325–8.

13.   Lantos P., and Wormser G. "Chronic Coinfections in Patients Diagnosed with Chronic Lyme Disease: A Systematic Review." *The American Journal of Medicine* 127.11 (2014): 1105–110.

14.   Nadelman R., and Wormser G. "Reinfection in Patients with Lyme Disease." *Clinical Infectious Diseases* 45.8 (2007): 1032–8.

15.   Nelson D., Bradley J., Ayra R., Merlin M., Ianosi-Irimie M., and Marques-Baptista A. "Babesiosis as a Rare Cause of Fever in the Immunocompromised Patient: A Case Report." *Cases Journal* 2 (2009): 7420.

16. Strie F., Cimperman J., Lotric-Furlan S., Maraspin V., and Ruzic-Sablijic E. "Rythema Migrans in the Immunocompromised Host." *Wien Klin Wochenschr* 111.22–23 (1999): 923–32.

17. Shoemaker R., Schaller J., and Schmidt P. *Mold Warriors: Fighting America's Hidden Health Threat.* Baltimore, MD: Gateway, 2005.

18. Teichman K. "Indoor Air Quality: Research Needs" *Occupational Medicine* 10.1 (1995): 217–27.

19. Corrier D. "Mycotoxicosis: Mechanisms of Immunosuppression." *Veterinary Immunology and Immunopathology* 30.1 (1991): 73–87.

20. Ngampongsa S., Hanafusa M., Ando K., Ito K., Kuwahara M., Yamamoto Y., Yamashita M., Tsuru Y., and Tsubone H. "Toxic Effects of T-2 Toxin and Deoxynivalenol on the Mitochondrial Electron Transport System of Cardiomyocytes in Rats." *The Journal of Toxicological Sciences* 38.3 (2013): 495–502.

21. Wang J., and Groopman J. "DNA Damage by Mycotoxins." *Mutation Research* 424 July 29, 1998: 167–81. http://toxicology.usu.edu/endnote/04302008004.pdf.

22. Tian J., Yan J., Wang W., Zhong N., Tian L., Sun J., Min Z., Ma J., and Lu S. "T-2 Toxin Enhances Catabolic Activity of Hypertrophic Chondrocytes through ROS-NF-κB-HIF-2α Pathway." *Toxicology in Vitro* 26.7 (2012): 1106–13.

23. Doi K., and Uetsuka K. "Mechanisms of Mycotoxin-Induced Neurotoxicity through Oxidative Stress-Associated Pathways." *International Journal of Molecular Sciences* 12.8 (2011): 5213–37.

24. Karunasena E. "The Mechanisms of Neurotoxicity Induced by a Stachybotrys Chartarum Trichothecene Mycotoxin in an in Vitro Model." Dissertation, Texas Tech University (2005): 1–115.

25. National Center for Immunization and Respiratory Diseases, Centers for Disease Control and Prevention. "About Epstein-Barr Virus (EBV) and Infectious Mononucleosis." September 14, 2016. http://www.cdc.gov/epstein-barr/about-mono.html.

26. Brisson D., Baxamusa N., Schwartz I., and Wormser G. "Biodiversity of Borrelia Burgdorferi Strains in Tissues of Lyme Disease Patients." *PLOS ONE* 6.8 (August 4, 2011). https://www.ncbi.nlm.nih.gov/pmc/articles/PMC3150399/.

27. US Food and Drug Administration. "FDA Public Health Advisory: Assays for Antibodies to Borrelia Burgdorferi; Limitations, Use, and Interpretation for Supporting a Clinical Diagnosis of Lyme Disease." *Public Health Notifications*, July 7, 1997. Last revised October 20, 2015. http://www.fda.gov/MedicalDevices/Safety/AlertsandNotices/PublicHealthNotifications/ucm062429.htm.

28. Salinas-Carmona M., Pérez L., Galán K., and Vázquez A. "Immunosuppressive Drugs Have Different Effect on B Lymphocyte Subsets and IgM Antibody Production in Immunized BALB/c Mice." *Autoimmunity* 42.6 (2009): 537–44.

29. Berghoff W. "Chronic Lyme Disease and Co-infections: Differential Diagnosis." *The Open Neurology Journal* 6.1 (2012): 158–78.

30. Garcia-Monco J., Frey H., Villar B., Golightly M., and Benach J. "Lyme Disease Concurrent with Human Immunodeficiency Virus Infection." *American Journal of Medicine* 87.3 (1989) 325–8.

31. Fallon B., and Nields J. "Lyme Disease: A Neuropsychiatric Illness." *American Journal of Psychiatry* 151.11 (1994): 1571–83.

32. Thomas J., and Posey S. "Biofilms Made Easy: A Picture Tutorial. Understanding the Impact of Microbiology, 'Focusing' on Biofilms." (2015): 1–54. https://www.yumpu.com/en/document/view/11732405/biofilms-made-easy-a-picture-tutorial-west-virginia-university-.

33. Center for Biofilm Engineering, Montana State University. "Biofilm Basics: What Are Biofilms?"Accessed April 17, 2015. http://www.biofilm.montana.edu/node/2390.

34. Høiby N., Ciofu O., and Bjarnsholt T. "Pseudomonas Aeruginosa Biofilms in Cystic Fibrosis." *Future Microbiology* 5.11 (2010): 1663–74.

35. Hall-Stoodley L., Hu F., Gieseke A., Nistico L., Nguyen D., Hayes J., Forbes M., Greenberg D., Dice B., Burrows A., Wackym P., Stoodley P., Post J., Ehrlich G.,and Kerschner J. "Direct Detection of Bacterial Biofilms on the Middle Ear Mucosa of Children with Chronic Otitis Media." *Journal of the American Medical Association* 296.2 (2006): 202–11.

36. Anderson G., Palermo J., Schilling J., Roth R., Heuser J., and Hultgren S. "Intracellular Bacterial Biofilm-Like Pods in Urinary Tract Infections." *Science* 301 (2003): 105–7.

37. Bendouah Z., Barbeau J., Hamad W., and Desrosiers M. "Biofilm Formation by Staphylococcus aureus and Pseudomonas aeruginosa is Associated with an Unfavorable Evolution after Surgery for Chronic Sinusitis and Nasal Polyposis." *Otolaryngology Head Neck Surgery* 134 (2006): 991–6.

38. Costerton J., Stewart P., and Greenberg E. "Bacterial Biofilms: A Common Cause of Persistent Infections." *Science* 284 (1999): 1318–22.

39. Parsek M., and Singh P. "Bacterial Biofilms: An Emerging Link to Disease Pathogenesis." *Annual Review of Microbiology* 57 (2003): 677–701.

40. Mohamed J., and Huang D. "Biofilm Formation by Enterococci." *Journal of Medical Microbiology* 56.12 (2007): 1581–8.

41. Chiaraviglio L., Duong S., Brown D., Birtles R., and Kirby J. "An Immunocompromised Murine Model of Chronic Bartonella Infection." *The American Journal of Pathology* 176.6 (2010): 2753–63.

42. Martinez L., and Fries B. "Fungal Biofilms: Relevance in the Setting of Human Disease." *Current Fungal Infection Reports* 4.4 (2010): 266–75.

43. Miller W. *The Microcosm Within: Evolution and Extinction in the Hologenome*. Boca Raton, FL: Universal Publishers, 2013, p. 81.

44. Petrova O., and Sauer K. "Sticky Situations: Key Components That Control Bacterial Surface Attachment." *Journal of Bacteriology* 194.10 (2012): 2413–25.

45. Hunt S., Werner E., Huang B., Hamilton M., and Stewart P. "Hypothesis for the Role of Nutrient Starvation in Biofilm Detachment." *Applied and Environmental Microbiology* 70.12 (2004): 7418–25.

46. Kalia V., Wood T., and Kumar P. "Evolution of Resistance to Quorum-Sensing Inhibitors." *Microbial Ecology* 68.1 (2013): 13–23.

47. Hernández-Jiménez E., Campo R., Toledano V., Vallejo-Cremades M., Muñoz A., Largo C., Arnalich F., García-Rio F., Cubillos-Zapata C., and López-Collazo E. "Biofilm vs. Planktonic Bacterial Mode of Growth: Which Do Human Macrophages Prefer?" *Biochemical and Biophysical Research Communications* 441.4 (2013): 947–52.

48. Costerton J., Lewandowski Z., Caldwell D., Korber D., and Lappin-Scott H. "Microbial Biofilms." *Annual Review of Microbiology* 49 (1995): 711–45.

49. Romanova I, and Gintsburg A. "Bacterial Biofilms as a Natural Form of Existence of Bacteria in the Environment and Host Organism." *Mikrobiology Epidemiology Immunobiology* 3 (2011): 99–109.

50. Romanova I., Didenko L., Tolordava E., and Gintsburg A. "Biofilms of Pathogenic Bacteria and Their Role in Chronization of Infectious Process: The Search for the Means to Control Biofilm." *Vestnik Rosillskoi Akademi Meditsinskikh Nauk.* 10 (2011): 31–9.

51. Høiby N., Ciofu O., Johansen H., Song Z., Moser C., Jensen P., Molin S., Givskov M., Nielsen T., and Bjarnsholt T. "The Clinical Impact of Bacterial Biofilms." *International Journal of Oral Science* 3.2 (2011): 55–65.

52. Macedo A., and Abraham W. "Can Infectious Biofilm Be Controlled by Blocking Bacterial Communication?" *Medicinal Chemistry* 5.6 (2009): 517–28.

53. Abraham W. "Controlling Biofilms of Gram-Positive Pathogenic Bacteria." *Current Medicinal Chemistry* 13.13(2006): 1509–24.

54. Kalia V. "Quorum Sensing Inhibitors: An Overview." *Biotechnology Advances* 31.2 (2013): 222–3.

55. Landini P., Antoniani D., Burgess J., and Nijland R. "Molecular Mechanisms of Compounds Affecting Bacterial Biofilm Formation and Dispersal." *Applied Microbiology and Biotechnology* 86.3 (2010): 813–23.

56. Anderson G., and O'Toole G. "Innate and Induced Resistance Mechanisms of Bacterial Biofilms." *Current Topics in Microbiology and Immunology Bacterial Biofilms* 322.85 (2008): 85–105.

57. Costerton J., Stewart P., and Greenberg E. "Bacterial Biofilms: A Common Cause of Persistent Infections." *Science* 284.5418 (1999): 1318–22.

58. Lewis K. "Multidrug Tolerance of Biofilms and Persister Cells." *Current Topics in Microbiology and Immunology Bacterial Biofilms* 322 (2008): 107–31.

59. Høiby B., Johansen H., Ciofu O., Jensen P., Bjarnholt T., and Givskov M. "Foreign Body Infections: Biofilms and Quorum Sensing." *Ugeskrit for Laeger* (2007): 4163–66.

60. Venkatesan N., Perumal G., and Doble M. "Bacterial Resistance in Biofilm-Associated Bacteria." *Future Microbiology* 10.11 (2015): 1743–50.

61. Zhang Q., Bos J., Tarnopolsky G., Sturm J., Kim H., Pourmand N., Austin R. "You Cannot Tell a Book by Looking at the Cover: Cryptic Complexity in Bacterial Evolution"*Biomicrofluidics*. 8.5 September 9 2014. http://scitation.aip.org/content/aip/journal/bmf/8/5/10.1063/1.4894410.

62. Usmani-Brown S., Halperin J., and Krause P. "Neurological Manifestations of Human Babesiosis." *Neuroparasitology and Tropical Neurology Handbook of Clinical Neurology* (2013): 199–203.

63. Vannier E., Gewurz B., and Krause P. "Human Babesiosis." *Infectious Disease Clinics of North America* 22.3 (2008): 469–88.

64. World Health Organization. "10 Facts on Malaria." November 2015. Accessed April 2, 2016 http://www.who.int/features/factfiles/malaria/en/.

65.   Marinella M. "Jarisch-Herxheimer Reaction." *Western Journal of Medicine* 165.3 (1996): 161–2.

66.   Belum G., Belum V., Chaitanya Arudra S., and Reddy B. "The Jarisch-Herxheimer Reaction: Revisited." *Travel Medicine and Infectious Disease* 11.4 (2013): 231–7.

67.   Mahabir S., Wei Q., Barrera S., Dong Y., Etzel C., Spitz M., and Forman M. "Dietary Magnesium and DNA Repair Capacity as Risk Factors for Lung Cancer." *Carcinogenesis* 29.5 (2008): 949–56.

68.   Hollmann M., Liu H., Hoenemann C., Liu W., and Durieux M. "Modulation of NMDA Receptor Function by Ketamine and Magnesium, Part II: Interactions with Volatile Anesthetics." *Anesthesia and Analgesia* 92.5 (2001): 1182–91.

69.   Ko Y., Hong S., and Pedersen P. "Chemical Mechanism of ATP Synthase: Magnesium Plays a Pivotal Role in Formation of the Transition State Where ATP is Synthesized from ADP and Inorganic Phosphate." *Journal of Biological Chemistry* 274.41 (1999): 28853–6.

70.   Zittermann A. "Magnesium Deficit: Overlooked Cause of Low Vitamin D Status?" *BMC Medicine* 11.1 (2013): 229.

71.   Sigma-Aldrich. "Mechanism of Action: Antibiotics." Accessed February 25, 2016. http://www.sigmaaldrich.com/life-science/biochemicals/bio-chemical-products.html?TablePage=14837959.

72.   Rafii F., Sutherland J., and Cerniglia C. "Effects of Treatment with Antimicrobial Agents on the Human Colonic Microflora." *Therapeutics and Clinical Risk Management* 4.6 (2008): 1343–58.

73. Grill M., and Maganti R. "Neurotoxic Effects Associated with Antibiotic Use: Management Considerations." *British Journal of Clinical Pharmacology* 72.3 (2011): 382–93.

74. Angelakis E., Million M., Kankoe S., Lagier J., Giorgi F., and Raoult D. "Abnormal Weight Gain and Gut Microbiota Modifications Are Side Effects of Long-Term Doxycycline and Hydroxychloroquine Treatment." *Antimicrobial Agents and Chemotherapy* 58.6 (2014): 3342–47.

75. Rapin J., and Wiernsperger N. "Possible Links between Intestinal Permeablity and Food Processing: A Potential Therapeutic Niche for Glutamine." *Clinics* 65.6 (2010): 635–43.

76. Ampting M., Van T., Schonewille A., Vink C., Brummer R., Van Der Meer R., and Bovee-Oudenhoven I. "Damage to the Intestinal Epithelial Barrier by Antibiotic Pretreatment of Salmonella-Infected Rats Is Lessened by Dietary Calcium or Tannic Acid." *Journal of Nutrition* 140.12 (2010): 2167–72.

77. Nanri K., Shibuya M., Taguchi T., Hasegawa A., and Tanaka N. "Selective Loss of Purkinje Cells in a Patient with Anti-gliadin-antibody-positive Autoimmune Cerebellar Ataxia." *Diagnostic Pathology* 6.1 February 4, 2011. https://www.ncbi.nlm.nih.gov/pmc/articles/PMC3042899/.

78. Trivedi M., Shah J., Al-Mughairy S., Hodgson N., Simms B., Trooskens G., Criekinge W., and Deth R. "Food-Derived Opioid Peptides Inhibit Cysteine Uptake with Redox and Epigenetic Consequences." *The Journal of Nutritional Biochemistry* 25.10 (2014): 1011–18.

79. Josephson R., Silverman H., Stern M, Lakatta E., and Zweier J. "Study of the Mechanisms of Hydrogen Peroxide and Hydroxyl Free

Radical–Induced Cellular Injury and Calcium Overload in Cardiac Myocytes." *Journal of Biological Chemistry* 266.4 (1991): 2354–61.

80. Mikarova N., Jackson J., and Riordan N. "The Effect of High Dose IV Vitamin C on Plasma Antioxidant Capacity and Level of Oxidative Stress in Cancer Patients and Healthy Subject." *Journal of Orthomolecular Medicine* 22.3 (2007): 153–60.

81. Mesiwala A., Farrell L., Santiago P., Ghatan S., and Silbergeld D. "The Effects of Hydrogen Peroxide on Brain and Brain Tumors." *Surgical Neurology* 59.5 (2003): 398–407.

82. Driessens N., Versteyhe S., Ghaddhab C., Burniat A., Deken X., Van Sande J., Dumont J., Miot F., and Corvilain B. "Hydrogen Peroxide Induces DNA Single- and Double-Strand Breaks in Thyroid Cells and Is Therefore a Potential Mutagen for This Organ." *Endocrine Related Cancer* 16.3 (2009): 845–56.

83. Filho A., Hoffmann M., and Meneghini R. "Cell Killing and DNA Damage by Hydrogen Peroxide Are Mediated by Intracellular Iron." *Biochemical Journal* 218.1 (1984): 273–75.

84. Koh C., Sam C., Yin W., Tan L., Krishnan T., Chong Y., and Chan K. "Plant-Derived Natural Products as Sources of Anti-Quorum Sensing Compounds." *Sensors* 13.5 (2013): 6217–228.

85. Dedeoglu F. "Drug-Induced Autoimmunity." *Current Opinion in Rheumatology* 21.5 (2009): 547–51.

86. Merz B. "Benzodiazepine Use May Raise Risk of Alzheimer's Disease." Harvard Health Blog, Harvard University, December 8 2015. http://www.health.harvard.edu/blog/benzodiazepine-use-may-raise-risk-alzheimers-disease-201409107397.

87.   Xiao X., and Chang C. "Diagnosis and Classification of Drug-Induced Autoimmunity (DIA)." *Journal of Autoimmunity* 48–49 (2014): 66–72.

88.   Mongey A., and Hess E. "Drug Insight: Autoimmune Effects of Medications—What's New?" *Nature Clinical Practice Rheumatology* 4.3 (2008): 136–44.

89.   Schüle, C. "Neuroendocrinological Mechanisms of Actions of Antidepressant Drugs." *Journal of Neuroendocrinology* 19.3 (2007): 213–26.

90.   Moncek F., Duncko R., and Jezova D. "Repeated Citalopram Treatment but Not Stress Exposure Attenuates Hypothalamic-Pituitary-Adrenocortical Axis Response to Acute Citalopram Injection." *Life Sciences* 72.12 (2003): 1353–65.

91.   Jensen J., Mørk A., and Mikkelsen J. "Chronic Antidepressant Treatments Decrease Pro-Opiomelanocortin MRNA Expression in the Pituitary Gland: Effects of Acute Stress and 5-HT1A Receptor Activation." *Journal of Neuroendocrinology* 13.10 (2008): 887–93.

92.   Visentin G., and Liu C. "Drug-Induced Thrombocytopenia." *Hematology/Oncology Clinics of North America* 21.4 (2007): 685–96.

93.   Hua J., Liang Q., Chen .T., and Wang X. "Resveratrol Protects Chondrocytes from Apoptosis via Altering the Ultrastructural and Biomechanical Properties: An AFM Study." *PLOS ONE* 9.3 March 14, 2014.   http://journals.plos.org/plosone/article?id=10.1371%2Fjournal.pone.0091611

94.   Dominguez R., and Holmes K. "Actin Structure and Function." *Annual Review of Biophysics* 40 (2011): 169–86.

95. Purves, D., Augustine G., Fitzpatrick D., Hall W., Lamantia A., McNamara J., and Williams S. "Neurotransmitters, Receptors, and Their Effects." in *Neuroscience, 3rd Ed.* Sunderland, MA: Sinauer Associates, Inc., 2004, pp. 129–65.

96. Limbrick, D., Sombati S., and DeLorenzo R. "Calcium Influx Constitutes the Ionic Basis for the Maintenance of Glutamate-Induced Extended Neuronal Depolarization Associated with Hippocampal Neuronal Death." *Cell Calcium* 33.2 (2003): 69–81.

97. Schmidt C. "Questions Persist: Environmental Factors in Autoimmune Disease." *Environmental Health Perspectives* 119.6 (2011): 248–53.

98. Cojocaru M, Cojocaru I, and Silosi I. "Multiple Autoimmune Syndrome." *Maedica Journal of Clinical Medicine* 5.2 (2010): 132–4.

99. Pavlov V., and Tracey K. "The Vagus Nerve and the Inflammatory Reflex: Linking Immunity and Metabolism." *Nature Reviews Endocrinology* 8.12 (2012): 743–54.

    Andersson U., and Tracey K. "Neural Reflexes in Inflammation and Immunity." *The Journal of Experimental Medicine* 209.6 (2012): 1057–68.

    Shoemaker, R. "The Biotoxin Pathway." 2011. Accessed March 20, 2014. http://www.consciouslivingcenter.com/images/BiotoxinPathway.jpg.

100. University of Minnesota, Environmental Health Sciences. "Indoor Molds: Absorption, Distribution, Metabolism, and Associated Sites of Toxicity of Molds." 2015. Accessed March 27, 2014. http://enhs.umn.edu/current/5103/molds/absorption.html.

101. US Food and Drug Administration. "Data on Benzene in Soft Drinks and Other Beverages." March 25, 2015. http://www.fda.gov/Food/FoodborneIllnessContaminants/ChemicalContaminants/ucm055815.htm.

102. Behrens M., Hüwel S., Galla H., and Humpf H. "Blood-Brain Barrier Effects of the Fusarium Mycotoxins Deoxynivalenol, 3 Acetyldeoxynivalenol, and Moniliformin and Their Transfer to the Brain." *PLOS ONE* 10.11 November 23, 2015. http://journals.plos.org/plosone/article?id=10.1371/journal.pone.0143640.

103. Wijnands L., and Van Leusden F. "An Overview of Adverse Health Effects Caused by Mycotoxins and Bioassays for Their Detection." *National Institute of Public Health and Environment* (2000): 2–99.

104. Ezra N., Dang K., and Heuser G. "Improvement of Attention Span and Reaction Time with Hyperbaric Oxygen Treatment in Patients with Toxic Injury Due to Mold Exposure." *European Journal of Clinical Microbiology and Infectious Disease* 30.1 (2010): 1–6.

105. Rocha O., Ansari K., and Doohan F. "Effects of Trichothecene Mycotoxins on Eukaryotic Cells: A Review." *Food Additives and Contaminants* 22.4 (2006): 369–78.

106. Bin-Umer M., McLaughlin J., Basu D., McCormick S., and Tumer N. "Trichothecene Mycotoxins Inhibit Mitochondrial Translation: Implication for the Mechanism of Toxicity." *Toxins* 3.12 (2011): 1484–501.

107. Pinton P., and Oswald I. "Effect of Deoxynivalenol and Other Type B Trichothecenes on the Intestine: A Review." *Toxins* 6.5 (2014): 1615–43.

108. Wong S., Schwartz R., and Pestka J. "Superinduction of TNF-α and IL-6 in Macrophages by Vomitoxin (Deoxynivalenol) Modulated by MRNA Stabilization." *Toxicology* 161.1–2 (2001): 139–49.

109. Wannemacher R., and Weiner S. "Trichothecene Mycotoxins" in *Medical Aspects of Chemical and Biological Warfare*. Washington, DC: TMM Publications, 1998, 655–76.

110. Kuhn D., and Ghannoum M. "Indoor Mold, Toxigenic Fungi, and Stachybotrys Chartarum: Infectious Disease Perspective." *Clinical Microbiology Reviews* 16.1 (2003): 144–72.

111. Bennett J., and Klich M. "Mycotoxins." *Clinical Microbiology Reviews* 16.3 (2003): 497–516.

112. Brewer J., Thrasher J., and Hooper D. "Chronic Illness Associated with Mold and Mycotoxins: Is Naso-Sinus Fungal Biofilm the Culprit?" *Toxins* 6.1 (2013): 66–80.

113. Verma Y., and Rana S. "Biochemical Toxicity of Benzene." *Journal of Environmental Biology* 2 (2005): 157–68.

114. Verma Y., and Rana S. "Modulation of Phase-II Enzymes Activities by Ovariectomy in Liver and Kidney of Benzene Treated Rats." *Environmental Toxicolgy and Pharmacology* 21.3 (2011): 371–7.

115. Yardley-Jones A., Anderson D., and Parke D. "The Toxicity of Benzene and Its Metabolism and Molecular Pathology in Human Risk Assessment." *British Journal of Industrial Medicine* 48.7 (1991): 437–44.

116. Donald J., Hooper K., and Hopenhayn-Rich C. "Reproductive and Developmental Toxicity of Toluene: A Review." *Environmental Health Perspectives* 94 (1991): 237–44.

117. Tchounwou P., Yedjou C., Patlolla A., and Sutton D. "Heavy Metals Toxicity and the Environment." *Molecular, Clinical and Environmental Toxicology* 101 (2012): 133–64.

118. Middleton F., and Strick P. "Basal Ganglia and Cerebellar Loops: Motor and Cognitive Circuits." *Brain Research Reviews* 31.2–3 (2000): 236–50.

119. Centers for Disease Control and Prevention, National Center for Emerging and Zoonotic Infectious Diseases. "Post-Treatment Lyme Disease Syndrome." July 1, 2015. http://www.cdc.gov/lyme/postlds/.

120. US Food and Drug Administration. "Hyperbaric Oxygen Therapy: Don't be Misled." May 10, 2016. http://www.fda.gov/ForConsumers/ConsumerUpdates/ucm364687.htm.

Made in the USA
San Bernardino, CA
10 May 2017